THE CARRIERS

THE CARRIERS

What the Fragile X Gene Reveals
About Family, Heredity,
and Scientific Discovery

ANNE SKOMOROWSKY

Foreword by Randi J. Hagerman, MD

Columbia University Press
New York

Columbia University Press
Publishers Since 1893
New York   Chichester, West Sussex
cup.columbia.edu

Library of Congress Cataloging-in-Publication Data

Names: Skomorowsky, Anne, author.
Title: The carriers : what the fragile X gene reveals about family,
heredity, and scientific discovery / Anne Skomorowsky.
Description: New York : Columbia University Press, [2022] |
Includes bibliographical references and index.
Identifiers: LCCN 2021034141 (print) | LCCN 2021034142 (ebook) |
ISBN 9780231197663 (hardback) |
ISBN 9780231552288 (ebook)
Subjects: MESH: Fragile X Syndrome—complications | Fragile X
Syndrome—genetics | Genetic Predisposition to Disease |
Heterozygote | Chromosome Fragile Sites—genetics
Classification: LCC RJ506.F73 (print) | LCC RJ506.F73 (ebook) |
NLM QS 677 | DDC 618.92/858841—dc23

Cover design: Henry Sene Yee

CONTENTS

CONTENTS

FOREWORD

I LOVE this book because it is the first in the lay literature to put together the multigenerational impact that we see from fragile X mutations, particularly the premutation. As one mother said to me, "I can't believe that just a small expansion of CGG repeats can cause so many problems." Well, I believe it, because I have seen these problems so very many times in the carriers that I have evaluated over many years. Some carriers do fine and have no problems, but many others suffer significantly from the toxic effects of too much mRNA and this expanded CGG repeat number.

This book is needed because too many doctors and other healthcare providers do not realize the problems associated with the premutation, and they often have it mixed up with the full mutation. The premutation is common in the general population: 1 in 150 women and 1 in 250 to 400 men have it, so doctors in all fields of medicine will see these patients, and if they do not test for it they will not know that the premutation may be causing the problems that the patient is experiencing.

I have heard from patients with the fragile X–associated tremor/ataxia syndrome (FXTAS) that their doctors comment about how they seem more intelligent than what they expected from fragile X syndrome (FXS). And when I read their medical reports, those doctors state that the patient has FXS when the problem is very different—specifically, FXTAS. So the confusion persists, and more literature, including lay publications, is needed.

This book fits that need. Most important, it is written by an intuitive psychiatrist who is very knowledgeable about emotional and personality issues related to the premutation, which affects her own family. Her analytical observations and honest critiques are hard to read sometimes, and many carriers may find them hard to absorb, since they strike so close to home. I had to work on digesting what she said about my husband and me, but it is all fair, and there are important truths in what she says. Anne Skomorowsky weaves in history about genetics and the discoveries of fragile X advances and research seamlessly with intense descriptions of the families that have human interest for everyone, so you will not put her book down because of boredom.

Too much of medicine is compartmentalized, even within the field of neurology. For instance, the headache doctor who sees a carrier for migraines does not necessarily communicate with the neurologist who sees her for neuropathy symptoms and the psychiatrist who sees the patient for anxiety or depression and makes a diagnosis not only of mood disorders but also of chronic pain. The clinicians usually do not think about how all of these problems are related to the premutation because on the reviews of etiologies for these disorders the premutation is not listed. Most lists for the etiology of intention tremor or cerebellar ataxia do not include the premutation and FXTAS, because this is a relatively newly described disorder known only since 2001. You would think that twenty years is time enough for this to be seen in medical textbooks, but it is not—another reason why such a book as this one is needed.

The story of the premutation is amazing. It weaves together hard science and molecular mechanisms with medical, neurological, and behavioral entities that clinicians in the past thought were completely separated. The premutation represents a broad group of disorders that unify medicine and psychiatry and challenge clinicians to think of new avenues of treatment. We are in an age of molecular interventions, specifically targeted treatments that may reverse the neurobiological abnormalities seen both in neurodevelopmental disorders including fragile X syndrome and in neurodegenerative disorders such as Parkinson's disease and FXTAS.

Coming close on the heels of targeted treatments are stem cell and gene therapy interventions that will change the face of medicine. Even today, mesenchymal cells from the placenta can reverse ovarian failure from chemotherapy and are likely a future treatment for FXPOI. New antisense oligonucleotides may eliminate excess mRNA in carriers. New medications such as ANAVEX 2-73 may eliminate the mitochondrial problems and oxidative stress in FXTAS and may even be preventative for developing FXTAS. The future of this field is exciting, as is medicine in general, and it is awaiting new clinician/investigators who will bring these new treatments to the patients. This book demonstrates the need for awareness of the fragile X spectrum disorders and will stimulate enthusiasm for this new area of research and discovery.

Randi J. Hagerman

INTRODUCTION

THE CARRIERS

THE PATELS were of South Asian descent, although all of the children had been born in New York.[1] The matriarch, Neha, over eighty years old, was crippled by arthritis. Her joints were like knobs on sticks. She had two daughters, Nina and Liz. Liz never spoke and never moved unless she had to. Nina was lively and handsome, with a big square face framed by a butch haircut, bouncy and irrepressible as a puppy. Unlike the two sisters, both of whom were in their late fifties, their older brother, Johnny, was frantic, disorganized, and unable to sit still.

Neha had managed the household and raised the children, but now that she was elderly and unable to get around, Nina had taken over. Nina could make lentils and rice and knew when to call 911, but she was too impulsive and childlike to run a home. Johnny victimized her, pinching and biting her when she tried to direct him. Finally, covered with bruises, she called for help.

The EMS workers who responded pronounced their apartment unfit to live in, and brought the entire family to the hospital, where their story emerged. The "children," now well into middle age, had never been educated. Because of Liz and Johnny's autism, none of them ever left home. It would have been too overwhelming for Liz and Johnny.

In the hospital, they were housed in a four-bed room, where each of them had a twin bed with its own TV. For the most part, they seemed pretty comfortable—except for Johnny. Although weeks went by as hospital officials tried to figure out what to do with the Patels, Johnny could not adjust to the new environment. Frequently, he ran out of his room, ripping his gown off, flying naked down hospital hallways through which elderly patients shuffled, clinging to IV poles. As a consulting psychiatrist, I was asked to prescribe medications to calm him.

Unfortunately, medications did not address Johnny's biggest problems. He was unable to express himself with words. He was incontinent; stool collected under his fingernails, but union regulations prohibited nurses from trimming them. Residential treatment centers would not accept him because he disrobed.

Given the family history—three children with intellectual disability, two of whom were autistic, one with severe anxiety—I suspected that fragile X was a likely possibility. Inherited via a tiny mutation on the X chromosome, one of the two paired chromosomes that determine a baby's sex, fragile X syndrome is characterized by intellectual disability, autism, emotional disturbance, and a distinctive appearance. Testing revealed that all three children had the full mutation, and Neha, their mother, was a carrier.

Neha had passed on the fragile X gene, and she had nurtured her family as long as she could. Nina, the least affected girl, had done her best to carry on. A team of sympathetic women—nurses, social workers, unit clerks, length-of-stay cops who looked the other way, non-union nail-trimmers hired by staff who had taken up a collection, and I as the attending psychiatrist—had assumed caregiving roles, but we had little to offer the Patels. Heavy sedation did make Johnny more tractable, and eventually the family was placed in a nursing home, where they were able to remain together for a time. Johnny returned to the hospital, this time alone, when his behavior decompensated again. This last hospital stay ended with rounds of intramuscular injections, restraints, and finally, aspiration pneumonia. He died in the intensive care unit before being reunited with his family.

In twenty years of practicing psychiatry, this was my first experience with fragile X syndrome.

■ ■ ■

A few years later, under very different circumstances, I encountered fragile X syndrome for a second time. In my private practice office a few miles from the hospital, I met Jessie for a consultation. Jessie had been on oral contraceptives for years, but when she went off the pill her period did not start up again.[2] Her doctor reassured her that this was not unusual, but months later she still was not menstruating and had begun to experience hot flashes. Hormone levels showed she had a condition called primary ovarian insufficiency—in lay terms, premature menopause. She was twenty-two.

Jessie's primary doctor referred her to a specialist in reproductive endocrinology who informed Jessie—wrongly, as it turned out—that there was only a 2 percent chance that she would ever have children. "It was such a heartbreaking shock for me," she told me during our first session. A petite, shy photographer who tended to hide behind a camera at parties, she began to avoid dating. She imagined that men wouldn't want to have anything to do with a woman who could not bear children.

Meanwhile, Jessie had noticed something. Her father had developed a tremor. Fortunately, it affected his nondominant hand, but he was increasingly anxious about it. What if it were Parkinson's disease? How could he continue to work as a surgeon if he could not control his own movements?

That Jessie's condition and her father's could be connected was a startling discovery. Jessie's endocrinologist ordered a genetic test to better evaluate her menopausal symptoms and in the process found an explanation for both her infertility and her father's tremor. A mutation on one of Jessie's X chromosomes known to scientists as *the fragile X premutation* put her at risk of passing on fragile X syndrome. Further testing of the family showed that she had inherited the mutation from her father.

But no one in Jessie's family is intellectually disabled. Jessie and her father did not have fragile X syndrome. They were carriers. Carriers of genetic diseases, by definition, should not be affected; they *carry* the disease to the next generation but do not suffer themselves. Over the past twenty-odd years, however, research has shown that fragile X is an exception. Jessie learned that she was never an unaffected carrier: the mutation had resulted in *fragile X–associated primary ovarian insufficiency* (FXPOI). Now it was causing her father to change as well.

The surgeon's tremor was an early sign of the *fragile X–associated tremor/ataxia syndrome* (FXTAS), a movement disorder that can progress to emotional displays, poor decision making, dementia, and death. (Ataxia is an abnormal gait in which the affected person sways and staggers as if drunk.) Jessie's father had noticed that he felt "tippy" when he got up too fast, though he walked normally. Jessie also saw that that little things such as soppy TV advertisements increasingly moved him to tears.

Jessie and her father each had a very different condition known to be associated with the fragile X carrier state. Going back a generation, Jessie's grandmother suffered from several complications that have been linked to the premutation: she fell frequently, had migraines and fibromyalgia, and went through menopause at thirty-five, and although she was witty and chic, she couldn't calculate a tip. Her grandmother's sister, eccentric and flamboyant, died childless in a one-car accident while still in her thirties, and Jessie's dad had always suspected suicide.

The unexpected diagnosis of a previously silent fragile X mutation had reframed an entire family's history. I wanted to know more.

A few minutes in the library pointed me to the work of Dr. Randi Hagerman and her colleagues at the Medical Investigations for Neurodevelopmental Disorders (MIND) Institute at the University of California, Davis. They had been studying the effects of the fragile X premutation on physical and mental health since it was discovered in the 1990s. They believed they could show that carriers had symptoms in multiple domains, and further, that the premutation was associated with certain personality traits. Looking over that research, it seemed to me that fragile X mutations could explain a lot of what Jessie had told me. The MIND Institute's researchers had a hypothesis: the fragile X premutation was *not* an asymptomatic carrier state. It was a group of disorders of a life-changing nature.

Although FXTAS typically begins in midlife or later, Randi Hagerman is a behavioral pediatrician, working in concert with geneticists and molecular biologists, including her husband, Paul Hagerman, their colleague Flora Tassone, and a genetic counselor, Louise Gane, at the MIND Institute. Often misdiagnosed as multiple sclerosis or Parkinson's disease, FXTAS is now a well-established consequence of the fragile X carrier state, but beyond that, it provides a model for how an invisible carrier state may affect psychological adjustment and physical health throughout the lifespan. As a psychiatrist who specializes in psychosomatic medicine—the study of the interplay of mind and body in disease—I was most intrigued by that question.

When I got to know the Hagermans, their colleagues, and others who have worked on fragile X syndrome since British geneticist Julia Bell first described it in the 1940s, I realized that premutation disorders were not only a fascinating medical mystery but also a window onto the special contributions of empathy, personality, and relationships in unraveling genetic disease. The tremor/ataxia syndrome and other conditions associated with the premutation were not discovered through technological innovations in a "Eureka" moment in a lab, but through caring and listening.

Without access to sophisticated technology to crack genetic codes, Julia Bell relied upon careful examination and inference to detect family patterns. In some ways a stereotypical Victorian spinster, Bell was intrigued by personal oddities, and she enjoyed uncovering evidence of lying and backstabbing. In describing families with genetic diseases, her primary tools were case collection, observation, and gossip. She paid attention to what women told her.

So did Randi Hagerman and her colleagues at the MIND Institute. Clinicians who worked with children with fragile X syndrome spent years developing relationships with their families as newly diagnosed infants grew up, and the trust that followed went both ways. Not only did the children's mothers speak freely to the researchers, but the researchers also respected the mothers as thoughtful observers of their families. When mothers began telling them that their fathers had developed symptoms like tremor, gait trouble, and personality changes, the MIND Institute's doctors took them seriously.

At Randi's invitation, I went to an international conference on the fragile X premutation in Sitges, Spain, in October 2015. I am accustomed to the American Psychiatric Association's annual meeting, which draws sixteen thousand psychiatrists, most of whom, frankly, rarely have anything new to say. In contrast, the premutation meeting comprised just eighty scientists at a seaside hotel. A major goal of the conference was to establish an international working group for the study of FXTAS. The researchers were there to define a new disease.

They showed film clips of older men with the tremor/ataxia syndrome singing and picking things up off the floor and of pre-mutation babies turning away from drawings of faces. They presented evidence that carriers had breast milk deficient in zinc, which could affect their babies from the moment they first latched on. They compared anxiety in mothers of children with fragile X syndrome with anxiety in mothers of children with autism of unknown cause. They were trying to understand something: What could be attributed to the fragile X premutation, and what had nothing to do with it?

This was the question I had begun to ask myself.

My search for understanding has taken me as far as India, where mothers of sons with fragile X syndrome hide their sons and their peculiar uncles from their daughters' suitors, and Colombia, where fragile X mutations traveled, like measles, with conquistadors from Spain. It has taken me to a dismal Ohio suburb, a Sacramento noodle joint, and the Centers for Disease Control in Atlanta. It has given me the privilege of speaking intimately with adults and children with fragile X syndrome and with their mothers and fathers. It has brought me to the library, the lab, and the bedside, where I have had the pleasure of learning alongside Randi Hagerman, her colleagues at the University of California, and other researchers from all over the world as they, too, try to understand how fragile X mutations affect us.

Like Julia Bell, I am intensely curious about unusual people. Their life histories, whether they are mundane or fit for tabloids, are what drew me to psychiatry. Whenever possible in researching this book, I use Bell's methods—tracking down families, traveling to meet them, observing individuals, collecting stories and documents, and allowing myself to be moved by the pathos and struggles they record.

Of necessity, much of my access to families has been made possible by Randi and her colleagues. This is a lively, curious group of people who do painstaking science with determination and joy. Though I have been swept up by their enthusiasm for all things fragile X, I have used scientific literature, my training as an academic psychiatrist, and my private observations to come to my own conclusions.

The Carriers asks how a tiny mutation on the X chromosome could affect character and fate but still remain invisible—until now. The mutation has shaped unsuspecting families for generations. It just needed time to make itself known.

■ ■ ■

Years ago, when I asked research psychologist David Hessl of the MIND Institute what he thought was the most important thing I could say to premutation carriers who might read this book, he said that he would want them to know that most premutation carriers are fully functional and have no overt deficits from their premutations.[3] But I have chosen to learn about those who *are* affected by the premutation, and it is these carriers—*patients*—who are the focus of my book.

Not every carrier is a patient or will ever be one. As an author, I have found it a challenge to balance the need to speak the truth on behalf of carriers who *are* patients with another truth: that many carriers are totally unaffected by the mutation.

Thus, I have presented some worst-case scenarios—entire families in disarray—and some in which a scare related to pre-natal testing is the worst thing a carrier will ever experience. I ask the reader to keep that balance in mind, too.

Chapter One

ONE DAMN THING AFTER ANOTHER

EVERY INDIVIDUAL has her own biography, but within families, our stories blend together, cross paths, and evolve in parallel. Each of the men and women of the Solitar family—four generations of one family in southern Ohio—has been affected by an undiagnosed genetic disease. We will see how their condition reveals itself in surprising ways as their narratives intersect and as a family saga takes a century to be told.

Please forgive me as I blurt out a diagnosis before even setting the scene of this medical mystery. The youngest generation of the Solitar family—Lina, who is now fifteen years old, and her brothers, Mike and Aaron, who are eighteen year-old identical twins—has fragile X syndrome, the most common known single-gene form of autism and intellectual disability. But this isn't their story. It is the story of their mother, their uncle, their grandmother, and their great-grandfather. These ancestors did not have fragile X syndrome: they were *carriers*. They may have looked like everybody else,

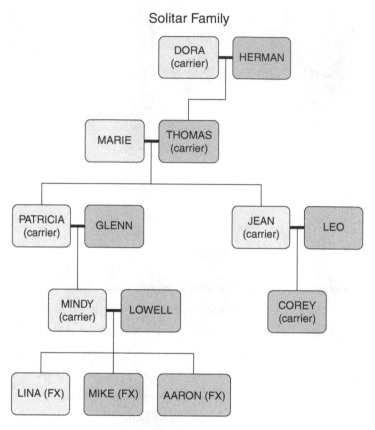

FIGURE 1.1 The Solitar family tree.

but carriers of the gene for fragile X syndrome—also known as *fragile X premutation carriers*—are different. Theirs is the true medical mystery.

Mike and Aaron are severely disabled, Lina less so. The three of them are what medical geneticists call *probands*, the first in their family to be diagnosed with an inherited disease. The diagnosis of fragile X syndrome provided closure for their parents, who sought an explanation for the kids' developmental delays and disturbed behavior. But when geneticists discover a proband, the story is just beginning. A proband opens the door to an entire family.

The Solitars had struggled with depression and anxiety, tremor, falls, dementia, infertility, chronic pain, autoimmune disease, drug addiction, and even a death by gunshot. They could never have guessed that these seemingly unrelated conditions had anything to do with fragile X syndrome. No one in the family had ever heard of it.[1]

COMPLICATIONS

Something was clearly wrong with the twins even before they were born. Their mother, Mindy, told me the story of her pregnancy and their early childhood as we split a donut at a Dunkin' Donuts just outside of Dayton, Ohio, in a strip mall between two suburban developments. One development had watered, green, neatly trimmed lawns overlooking a duck pond. Mindy had grown up there. The other was a worn-down version of the first. The houses needed fresh paint, and instead of a pond, there was a senior center that had closed and been allowed to decay. Kids played in the grass in front of the empty building.

This was where Mindy lived now, with her daughter and the twins and her husband, Lowell. Though I had come to Ohio to meet the Solitar family, Mindy did not invite me to her house. It was a mess, she said; she and the children had been ill. Our family visits took place in the pleasant neighborhood where Mindy's parents still lived in her childhood home. For privacy, Mindy and I met at Dunkin' Donuts.

Mindy wears loose clothes and is naturally feminine, without makeup or jewelry. Her long hair and healthy color make her look younger than forty-two. Appealingly unkempt in a hippie sundress, she reminded me, just a little, of Janis Joplin, with a hard edge that came out when she talked about what she and her children had been through. She called herself a "wallflower." But she was more like a flower child who had run into a wall.

As a teenager, Mindy did not flourish in the neat cul-de-sac where she grew up with stern, traditional parents who were often disappointed in her. She wanted to be a singer or an actress, but her parents did not approve of this ambition. She couldn't wait to get out of the house. When Mindy was eighteen, she found herself a minimum-wage job out of state and took off. She married young, at nineteen, and after a round of miscarriages, ovarian cysts, and a diagnosis of endometriosis, she became pregnant with twins.

It was a complicated pregnancy with several admissions to the hospital for intractable morning sickness and preterm labor. At twenty-eight weeks, she moved into the hospital to wait for the babies to come. At thirty-four weeks of gestation, Mindy noticed a strange sensation, as though one of the babies were shivering or seizing. Labor was urgently induced, and Mike and Aaron were rushed off to be resuscitated.

It turned out that the boys had twin-twin transfusion syndrome, a disease of the placenta, which is shared by identical twins. In twin-twin transfusion, the placenta directs the flow of blood from the mother to the babies unevenly. Aaron was nearly twice the size of his brother. Mike was undernourished and yellow from jaundice, while Aaron was fat and flushed from an excess of red blood cells. It took a month or so for the twins to stabilize, during which time they were in and out of the hospital.

When the boys finally settled into life at home, their first year was a trial. Mike in particular screamed day and night. They had to be persuaded to feed, and they gagged and threw up a lot. They were not interested in toys. Mike appeared to be deaf, whereas Aaron was terrified of noise. They rocked back and forth on their hands and knees but did not crawl, and they banged their heads deliberately. They didn't utter syllables until well after their first birthday.

Mindy and Lowell were quite concerned about the boys' development, but as you hear endlessly in parent stories about intellectual disability, the pediatrician told them not to worry. The boys were twins with birth complications. More diagnostic workup was not necessary.

But when the boys were two and a half years old, still unable to walk without holding on, with no meaningful words, Mindy gave birth to their sister, Lina. At the hospital, somebody thought that she might have Down syndrome, and a specialist was called in. Lina did not have Down syndrome, but the specialist noticed the twins, who were at their mother's bedside. They were engaged in play that Mindy and Lowell called "bear-cubbing"—rolling around together in a disorganized way, often biting and scratching each other. That didn't seem normal to the visiting specialist. The boys were evaluated for early intervention and given a diagnosis of "global developmental delay."

At first, baby sister Lina was a joy. Intellectually and physically, she was right on target. But as a toddler she rarely slept for more than a few hours, ran about constantly, and refused to be held. As she grew older she became aggressive and self-abusive. She used her verbal abilities to swear and argue. She was given a diagnosis of "oppositional defiant disorder"—a psychiatric term that really means bad behavior.

For many families the most distressing aspects of fragile X syndrome are behavioral and emotional. The mutation that causes fragile X syndrome interferes with habituation, the normal process by which we get used to noxious stimuli, so that we don't jump out of our skins, for example, at every single clap during a round of applause. Many individuals with fragile X syndrome never get comfortable with loud noises and other intrusions, even minor ones that most of us would not notice. Daily life can feel relentlessly stimulating.

That state of being flooded by unpleasant overstimulation is called *hyperarousal*, and it may be the defining experience of life with fragile X syndrome. It feels awful. To manage hyperarousal, people with fragile X syndrome may learn to avoid eye contact, shrink from being touched, and prefer familiar, safe routines. People with fragile X syndrome may engage in self-soothing behaviors like rocking and hand-flapping; on the other hand, they may instinctively defend themselves through impulsive, even assaultive behavior. When overstimulation reaches a tipping point, young people with fragile X syndrome may explode in a full-blown tantrum, during which they can destroy property, hurt themselves, and injure people they love.

In traditional psychiatric diagnostic terms, many fragile X kids have attention deficit hyperactivity disorder, and about 60 percent of boys meet full criteria for autism. Nearly all have autistic traits.

In many ways, Mike and Aaron were typical fragile X boys. They could be cuddly and giggly. Like many fragile X kids, they loved simple wordplay and cracked up over puns. They were obsessive fans of country music and professional wrestling. But they were intolerant of change, and anxiety could make them violent. Both boys had broken Mindy's nose and fingers during tantrums caused by the hyperarousal intrinsic to fragile X syndrome.

The fragile X diagnosis was not made until the children were school-aged. A TV show aired a segment about fragile X syndrome. It was eye-opening for Mindy and Lowell; it had never occurred to them that their kids' problems might have a genetic basis.

Mindy and Lowell returned to the pediatrician and asked for a genetic test. The test confirmed the diagnosis of fragile X syndrome in all three children. Lina was the least affected, but they all had what is known as the fragile X *full mutation*.

A FLIGHT FROM HELL

Though Mindy and Lowell were relieved to finally have a diagnosis established for their children, their household became still more chaotic as the kids grew older. At home, the boys threw furniture and beat each other and their sister. At school, they threw garbage cans and gave their teachers the finger. Mike, ten years old at the time, got into the family car and drove it until he crashed it in an alleyway.

The children never seemed to need any sleep. No matter how late it was, one child was always awake and in need of attention. If they weren't kept calm, they got on each other's nerves, precipitating outbursts. Lina infuriated her brothers by mimicking them.

Because of their tendency for hyperarousal, kids with fragile X syndrome are upset by conflict and may be frightened of being approached, even by family. With three fragile X kids acting up at home, someone was always being terrified and reacting with tantrums and aggression, which in turn terrified the next one. Both boys were admitted to psychiatric hospitals more than once, and each needed several medications for sleep and behavior.

The entire family was in crisis.

Mindy was desperate for help, but asking professionals to intervene brought only more grief. Unfamiliar with fragile X syndrome, authorities from the local developmental disability bureaucracy implied—without any foundation—that Mindy and Lowell might be abusing the children. (Otherwise, they suggested, why would the kids be so disturbed?) Recommendations that Mindy get psychological help, while they may have been well-intended, led to doctors' visits that left Mindy feeling vulnerable and misunderstood. As Mindy got angrier, so, it seemed, did the staff of the children's schools and others meant to look out for their best interests. It seemed to Mindy that some of the children's teachers truly disliked them for behaviors they could not control.

Then their pediatrician had an idea. She had been to a medical conference in Sacramento where a behavioral pediatrician, Dr. Randi Hagerman, had given a talk on fragile X syndrome. Hagerman was the medical director of the MIND Institute at the University of California, Davis. A leader in the field of intellectual and social disability in kids and a charismatic speaker, she was optimistic and had specific ideas about how to help fragile X children. Could Mindy get her family to the MIND for an evaluation by an expert?

The evaluation would be comprehensive, with psychological and IQ testing, radiologic studies, medical exams, and recommendations for treatment for the children. It would include more detailed genetic testing, not just for the children but for Mindy, her parents, and her grandparents. It would identify carriers and problems associated with the carrier state. The evaluation was free, but the family would bear the costs of travel.

It took over a year to make it happen. When the day finally came, there was an airport scene from hell as three hyperactive howling fragile X kids who had never flown before waited for a delayed flight along with their great-grandparents, who were in their nineties, and dozens of tense, disapproving fellow travelers. At the car rental area in Sacramento, Lina called 911 when she lost sight of her brothers for a moment. While her father and grandfather waited quietly at the car rental counter, police descended upon the airport.

Finally, they arrived at the MIND Institute.

TURNING DOWN THE VOLUME

For Mindy, at wit's end with her husband and kids, the visit to the MIND Institute was lifesaving. As a mother, she was flailing. She was desperate for a smart, empathic, authoritative clinician to provide direction. In Randi Hagerman, she found just that.

Randi had specific suggestions about routines and medications to help the kids settle. More important, she understood how incapacitating anxiety and hyperarousal can be in children and adults with full mutation fragile X syndrome. The children could not tolerate noise, emotional displays, and high-pitched voices that rose in anger or fear, all of which were daily occurrences in a tumultuous household. Randi showed Mindy and Lowell, pushed to their limits, how to turn down the volume. Decreasing overstimulation was the key to helping the children.

She also "got" Mindy. One of the ironies of the carrier state is that carrier mothers may be ill suited to care for children with intellectual disability and emotional disturbance. As a carrier with a premutation, Mindy, too, was easily overstimulated, anxious, and distractible. Self-effacing and often overwhelmed, Mindy found her own life humiliating. With her businesslike parents and innumerable educational bureaucrats constantly telling her what to do, Mindy was always on edge, feeling inadequate and ashamed. When I asked Mindy why the visit was so important to her, she explained that it freed her from relentless self-criticism. Randi had told her that she could not "fix" her kids; their difficulties were caused by fragile X syndrome.

Parenting wasn't the problem. Bossy special-ed case managers weren't the problem either. For her own sanity, she needed to stop fighting and blaming.

Randi advised Mindy to limit the number of people in her home and in her affairs, and to look inward, to take care of herself. As a fragile X premutation carrier, Mindy wasn't like everybody else. She needed to acknowledge that and ease up on herself.

Being diagnosed with the fragile X premutation helped Mindy see her struggles differently. She hadn't just passed a genetic disease to her children. She had one herself.

Looking back, Mindy believes that her own life has been dominated by fragile X, since way before the twins were born. At the MIND Institute, Mindy learned why this was biologically true. As an apparently unaffected carrier of fragile X syndrome, she was indeed different.

"She was a very difficult child to raise," her father told me without rancor, but firmly. As a little girl, Mindy was hyper-active, socially awkward, and anxious. She was unaware of her body in space, and often fell, hurt herself, and knocked things over. She has a big scar on her thigh from climbing up a cabinet and falling onto a coffee pot when she was five years old.

Mindy couldn't focus at school, couldn't do mathematics, and couldn't write a term paper that made sense. It was as though she had a mild case—just a whiff—of fragile X syndrome herself.

Mindy described her childhood self as "naïve." She was the girl who left a rose on the windshield of a popular boy's car with a love note that inevitably fell into the hands of her school-mates, to the great amusement of everyone but Mindy. She nursed dreams of stardom as a singer and dancer, and she got herself to New York City with a best friend without her parents' knowledge for an audition. Her parents still think the trip is a fantasy—in fact, they took me aside, embarrassed, to tell me that after she mentioned it in their presence—but I believe her. There is a lot that her parents don't know about Mindy.

She wasn't friendless, but her friends probably never knew how anxious and preoccupied with navigating social challenges she was. She couldn't get a read on other people, so she faked her way through social encounters, trying to behave appropriately without letting anyone see how scared she was.

I think that is why her parents felt Mindy was so difficult, though they couldn't come up with a single example of really untoward behavior. She was hyperactive and at times rude; she was klutzy and careless with her body; and she didn't excel in school the way two traditional parents might expect their bright child to do. But what really bothered them was that they didn't *know* Mindy. She didn't let them see inside her, because she was trying so hard not to look herself.

A TOUCH OF FRAGILE X

Mindy, her mother, and her maternal grandfather have symptoms that fall into three buckets, each of which I will discuss in more detail. The first bucket might be described as "a touch of fragile X syndrome." The second is related to a "toxic gain of function" of RNA, or RNA toxicity (about which more to come). And the third bucket is a collection of "anecdotal" associations—meaning, doctors have noticed the recurrence of these symptoms in carriers but don't yet have a good explanation for it.

Lina and the twins have full mutation fragile X syndrome: the mutation means that the boys cannot make the *fragile X mental retardation protein*, or FMRP, which is required for normal brain development. Lina, with one normal X chromosome, makes about 50 percent of the normal level. Mindy, a carrier, makes more FMRP than Lina, but as a mother of fragile X kids, with a significant premutation, she is not likely to make a normal level either.[2] She has enough to stave off fragile X syndrome, but her lower-than-normal FMRP level puts her at risk for what appear to be mild features of fragile X syndrome— putting her into the "a touch of fragile X syndrome" category. A few (rare) carriers have intellectual disability and are on the autism spectrum. More commonly, as is the case with Mindy, carriers may have difficulty picking up social cues and suffer from social anxiety, ADHD, learning disabilities, clumsiness, and disorganization.

Research suggests that there are subtle differences in personality in some carrier women. One study showed that carrier women were more likely to see standardized faces as "untrustworthy,"[3] and another showed that even carrier infants had very mild autistic behaviors.[4] Psychiatrist James Bourgeois, who studies the phenomenon, told me of an "avoidant, deferential character style" common to female carriers.[5] His opinion is based on personal experience, not established by scientific methods. But as a description of Mindy, it is spot-on.

"All my life, I was a wallflower. I felt I had to apologize all the time," Mindy told me. Perhaps that is what that psychiatrist meant by "avoidant and deferential." But I saw her—and many other carrier women whom I met while researching this book—somewhat differently: vague, shy, not quite able to articulate how she is feeling, and not quite able to hold her own at a party, a job, or even in her own family. She always thought she was doing something wrong.

At Dunkin' Donuts, Mindy confided that in her twenties she had had recurring nightmares about drowning. She told me that one night she walked to the piano while asleep, sat down, and played "Für Elise," Beethoven's haunting solo piano piece. She was so disturbed by this episode that she consulted a hypnotherapist to help her process it. In a hypnotic trance, she associated "Für Elise" with the last moments of the film *Titanic* (though "Für Elise" does not appear in the film). She saw herself in a blue gown, dancing as the ship sank.

That reminded me of something. When my daughter was about three years old, she loved *Alice in Wonderland*, the Disney cartoon. When I asked her what was so special about it, she said two words: "blue dress." At first I thought that for my daughter, Alice's sky-blue pinafore *represented* everything magical and exciting in Wonderland. But then I looked at it more literally, like a three-year-old would. That was some blue. You couldn't take your eyes off it.

Mindy thinks like that, too. She tells the story of her visit to the hypnotherapist as though it resolved a question, but there is no logic to it; if there *is* a narrative, it was borrowed from a movie. The gown, the waltz, the dirge, and the sinking ship were all intense—and frightening—sensory experiences. Of course, she was telling me about a dream. But it is my impression that dreaminess characterizes her waking life as well.

As the autistic author Temple Grandin puts it, many people on the spectrum don't think in words but in pictures.[6] What Mindy was describing wasn't a story; it was globs of sensory imagery, loosely stuck together.

When Mindy says that she couldn't write a coherent paper in high school, she is talking about her *mind*. Problems with attention, focus, and organization undermine her thinking. That is what I mean by "a touch of fragile X." It's as though her mind can't stand up for itself; it gets all wishy-washy and can't form a linear argument.

Such weaknesses could also make her susceptible to victimization.

Randi Hagerman's clinic notes from the Solitars' visit to the MIND Institute document this aspect of Mindy's history from a physician's perspective. All three of Mindy's children were violent as youngsters. Mike had clawed, punched, and even attempted to stab her by the time he was ten. He licked people, walls, and floors. Randi remarked that he ignored 90 percent of requests. At that same visit, Aaron was noted to spit and slap, and it was reported that he had broken Mindy's nose and beaten Lina with a stick. Mindy and Lowell could not set limits on their behavior, and when Mindy turned to the child welfare, special education, and mental health services for help, she was patronized, blamed, and bullied.

My own impression of Mindy's marriage is that it echoes her experience as a mother of children with special needs. Her husband is not abusive, but he does overwhelm with an incessant flood of speech, on any topic, regardless of whether anyone is listening. My impression is that Lowell copes through exhaustive online research and talking about his findings at length, which tends to add to the noise and chaos in the house rather than calm it. Mike delivers monologues about Shania Twain. Lowell delivers monologues about whatever topic is floating through his mind at the moment. Mindy isn't oblivious to his rambling, but she behaves as though she has no choice but to let the waves of speech flow over her.

Of course, Mindy is a stressed-out, impoverished mother of three challenging intellectually disabled teenagers, which would be overwhelming for anybody, and she is married to a stressed-out, impoverished man, a circumstance that is hardly confined to fragile X carriers. So what evidence is there that the fragile X carrier state has anything to do with Mindy's brain and body?

It takes four generations of Solitars to see how fragile X has shaped this family. So now I need to introduce Mindy's mother, Patricia, and move on from the "touch of fragile X" bucket to what is known as RNA toxicity: too much RNA in carriers.

RNA TOXICITY

Patricia is in her mid-seventies now, a small woman with fluffy short hair and big glasses, a look that hasn't changed much since she got married in the 1960s. When I visited the Solitars over a long weekend in May 2018, she wore a blue and green print shift that might have been in vogue back then, and it still looks just right on her. She is a retired bank teller, and her husband, Glenn, owns a restaurant supply store.

They live in a cute cul-de-sac in a dark and peaceful ranch house, with heavy brown furnishings. A boldly colored collection of sixteen Lady Diana dishes brightens the walls of the dining room.

Patricia doesn't like to complain, and you'd never guess she was in poor health if you came upon her sitting in a chair. She does have, however, a significant tremor and problems with balance and gait. She has some short-term memory loss. Her tremor affects her head and voice, so that she often sounds like she is holding back tears, even when she isn't.

Glenn tends to hover and keeps Patricia on track. When Patricia spoke of emotionally charged incidents—which she did, at my request—he deflected her kindly whenever she got too angry or seemed as if she might be about to blurt out a secret.

Patricia retired early from the bank, at fifty-five, because she had developed a hand tremor so severe that she could no longer handle money. She was embarrassed by her tremor and imagined that it was disturbing to her clients and coworkers. That was twenty years ago. Since then, Patricia has had problems with balance and walks unsteadily. She has had several serious falls and a hip fracture. But there was no explanation for the tremor and gait disturbance until Mindy brought the family to the MIND Institute.

Randi published the first paper on what she called *fragile X–associated tremor/ataxia syndrome* (FXTAS) in 2001.[7] (Ataxia, as we have noted, refers to an unsteady, weaving gait—how people walk when they are drunk.) Four years later, when

Patricia came to the MIND Institute with her family, the medical community was just beginning to acknowledge FXTAS as a legitimate neurologic diagnosis. It is now appreciated as an important degenerative neurologic disease associated not just with tremor and ataxia but also with loss of muscle strength, personality change, and dementia. People with full mutation fragile X syndrome don't develop these symptoms. Only carriers do.

The symptoms of FXTAS are caused by a "toxic gain of function" of RNA in carriers of fragile X syndrome. Briefly, the fragile X premutation, or carrier state, causes excess RNA to be produced. The surfeit of RNA traps proteins, which "pile on like a scrum in rugby," as molecular biologist Paul Hagerman puts it.[8] Proteins in clumps can no longer do their jobs, and the affected cells are inefficient.

Toxic RNA particularly damages the brain and the ovaries. FXTAS is something of a worst-case scenario for older carriers. Problems with daily living can be crippling, and behavioral issues can be heartrending for families.

And in *fragile X–associated primary ovarian insufficiency*, known by its acronym as FXPOI, RNA toxicity is hypothesized to damage the ovaries of young women, causing infertility and other reproductive problems. Patricia and Mindy both have symptoms of FXPOI. Both had ovarian cysts and menstrual irregularities. And both went through menopause before the age of forty.

FXTAS and FXPOI are best understood as *fragile X disorders*, a group that includes but is no longer limited to fragile X syndrome.

ANECDOTALLY . . .

There is a third category of symptoms associated with fragile X, and these are *anecdotal* associations. An anecdote, of course, is a little story, and anecdotal evidence in medicine might look like this: "I've seen three or four cases of thyroid disease in fragile X carriers in the past week," or, "If I went in for a hug, and a patient tried to kiss me, I knew he had FXTAS!"

While FXTAS and FXPOI are the most widely recognized complications of the premutation, Randi and her colleagues at the MIND Institute and other institutions have found, anecdotally, that a number of other medical and psychiatric conditions often cluster in carriers. In 2018, Randi began to call these conditions "FXAND."[9] The MIND Institute has conducted several studies showing an increased incidence of autoimmune disorders, sleep disorders, chronic pain syndromes, fibromyalgia, psychiatric disorders such as depression and anxiety, chronic fatigue, and hypertension in carriers.

Mindy has experienced multiple medical problems believed to be related to the fragile X carrier state. She has Crohn's disease, an autoimmune disease that affects the entire GI tract, type 2 diabetes mellitus, pelvic pain, chronic fatigue, and fibromyalgia. She had wanted to be a dancer, but the premutation gave her hyperextensible joints, which caused recurrent injuries and, subsequently, arthritis. Mindy is in pain every day. She can't stand or sit for long periods. To top that off, she is showing signs of FXTAS. Now that she is in her forties, she has a little tremor herself, and she often sounds like she is about to cry, even when she isn't.

Patricia also has a number of conditions anecdotally associated with the premutation, including rheumatoid arthritis, fibromyalgia, and neuropathy. She has obstructive sleep apnea. She experiences severe chronic fatigue and needs to sleep ten to twelve hours a night.

Psychiatrically, she has a long history of depression. She described herself as a "hoarder." (I saw no evidence of this, but Mindy assured me the hoard was upstairs, hidden from guests. Perhaps the royal family memorabilia marked the tip of an iceberg.) Patricia told me that she had a longstanding habit of twisting and pulling her hair.

Of course, conditions like anxiety and depression are so common that they are probably found in every family; however, surveys of fragile X carriers reveal higher-than-expected levels of distress, even when accounting for the stresses associated with caring for children with fragile X syndrome.

STILL THE FAMILY ROCK

More than a hundred years ago, Patricia's father, Thomas, was born in a small town in Indiana. When Patricia's father married, Patricia's mother took the story even farther into the past. She liked poking around in libraries and archives, and she researched the family's lineage as far back as the 1740s, long before their ancestors crossed the Atlantic from Germany and Scotland.

The scrapbook Patricia's mother, Marie, created is a marvel of historical evidence and dedication to detail. Its pages are decorated with early twentieth-century newspaper clippings of kids in crocheted dresses parading down Main Street, photos of brash college girls in Buddy Holly glasses and high collars, sober husbands standing beside smiling brides, and little children posing for Christmas portraits. Everything about this family is just *fine*.

What the family had no way of knowing was that Thomas and his ancestors were carriers of a fragile X mutation. Today, at 101 years of age, he is still the family rock, though he does suffer from tremor and is wheelchair-bound because of FXTAS. As a male carrier of a premutation on his X chromosome, he passed his X chromosome—and the premutation—to Patricia.

A FAMILY TRAGEDY

In 2015, researchers at the MIND Institute published a paper in the journal *Neurology*. It began:

> To our knowledge, we report the youngest deceased patient with FXTAS yet known. . . . His medical history included Asperger syndrome, restless legs syndrome, irritable bowel syndrome, type 2 diabetes mellitus, obesity, depression/anxiety, migraines, hypertension, and hypothyroidism, all associated with the premutation. He experienced handwriting problems, balance problems with frequent tripping and 2 falls in the previous year, and a slight postural tremor and an intention tremor in the head and right hand beginning in his late 20s.[10]

This was Corey, Mindy's first cousin. Corey's medical history, as shown here, was consistent with FXTAS, and his brain at autopsy showed the neuropathologic changes of FXTAS as well, confirming the diagnosis. In the paper, Corey's death was described as "an accident." But it was no accident.

Predictably, Corey was a carrier. Why predictably? Because his mother, Jean, was Patricia's sister. Jean and Patricia were *obligate* carriers. That means that because their father, Thomas, carried a premutation on his X chromosome, *all* his daughters were obliged to inherit it. Girls always get their fathers' X chromosomes.

The other thing about Corey's death that was not an accident? It was manslaughter.

Leo, Corey's father, shot Corey to death, allegedly in self-defense. Leo is the only living witness to the confrontation, but Corey's survivors were not surprised by the story his father told about the shooting. The men had been on a hunting trip during deer season in Michigan's Upper Peninsula. Leo went to the truck to get a steak for the barbecue. When he returned, he found Corey agitated, aggressive. Corey had threatened to kill his parents, Glenn told me, for drug money many times over many years. He was hooked on amphetamines.

Leo claimed he acted instinctively to save himself. He told the court that he believed that only one of them would survive the encounter. He shot Corey three times in the chest with his hunting rifle. (Leo was sentenced to four years in jail for the killing, but soon thereafter was released on partial parole.)[11]

Corey had been an awkward boy who was very lonely. Like Mindy, he was inattentive, active, and fell and hurt himself a lot as a child. Like Mindy, he was musically talented and wanted to perform, but unlike Mindy, he wasn't good-looking and sweet, and failure seemed certain. He had several tics. He was starving for friendship, and he especially longed for a girlfriend. Toward the end of high school, he started hanging out with boys who had, as Glenn put it, "no ambition." His friends grew up troubled, while the women in his life often took advantage of whatever money he had in hand. His vulnerabilities were likely to have made him more of a victim than a leader.

Mindy believes he turned to drugs to boost his confidence, but once he got involved with gang culture, he didn't have the street smarts to succeed. Far from fitting in as a would-be gangster, Mindy told me, he was tortured by alleged gang members. He dealt cocaine and methamphetamine, but he never seemed to have any money. He had two psychiatric hospitalizations and was diagnosed with bipolar disorder. Glenn, Mindy, and Thomas agree that he began to threaten to kill his mother, and even to threaten to have his friends kill her. (Jean declined to be interviewed for this book.)

A death like Corey's raises so many questions. It certainly had a multitude of possible factors. Corey was both a victim in death and a perpetrator—if indeed he threatened his mother's life—of domestic violence. He was addicted to drugs. He may have had bipolar disorder, though it is my impression that bipolar disorder is overdiagnosed in people who use stimulants.

His premutation put him at risk for FXTAS, and he developed it very young. It is suspected that exposure to poisons—stimulants, cocaine, alcohol—amplifies the damage caused by toxic RNA. In a vicious circle, developing FXTAS may have further impaired Corey's judgment. FXTAS is not just a movement disorder; it also affects the whole brain. In particular, it can cause memory impairment, impulsivity, indecisiveness, and difficulty with planning and organizing behavior. For a guy using and selling drugs, these weaknesses were a huge vulnerability. And the more Corey endured abusive relationships and social isolation, the more he depended on drugs and the money he needed to buy them.

Can Corey's death be connected to the premutation? Not definitively. But the fact that he had been diagnosed with Asperger syndrome and that social deficits played a prominent role in his life choices suggests to me that he may have had a neurodevelopmental disorder on the autism spectrum, in addition to anxiety that may have driven him to use drugs to self-medicate. Perhaps his autistic traits and inability to fit in were another case of "a touch of fragile X syndrome." In addition, RNA toxicity may have disrupted his early development—it is associated with autism spectrum disorders in a small number of premutation boys—as well as causing FXTAS. Glenn remembers noticing how odd he was when he was only five or six years old, long before drugs were in the picture. The combination of a developmental disorder and stimulant abuse accelerates the onset of FXTAS and was a recipe for an explosion.

Corey's death was not an accident. It was the result of a cascade of events that culminated in his being alone with a man with a gun, a man who happened to be his father, drinking beer before dinner with a stash of methamphetamine by his side. Could a genetic predisposition have played a role in his being in a particular frame of mind, with a particular personal history, at that place, at that time, with the person who killed him?

The research paper in *Neurology* makes that case from a scientific perspective; for Mindy, the answer is obvious. Her love for the sad little boy she grew up with, whose most memorable success was playing Daddy Warbucks in a grade-school musical, tells her that being amphetamine-addicted and shot dead was never a choice.

THE CARRIERS

I have chosen to write about the Solitars, an unusually severely affected fragile X family, because they show us how fragile X disorders can insinuate themselves throughout a family for generations before obviously impaired kids like Lina, Mike, and Aaron bring them into the laboratory for genetic testing. They were generous and brave enough to share their stories with a stranger.

Of course, every individual represents a unique outcome of genetic endowment and life experience, so for any particular family member, it may be difficult to see how fragile X mutations played a role. But with a family like the Solitars, one can look backward and notice a pattern that began to surface before World War I. Over time, the disturbance starts earlier, worsens, and eventually engulfs an entire generation. Thomas had a late-life onset of tremor and ataxia. His daughter, Patricia, had a midlife onset of the same, in addition to reproductive anomalies like early menopause. Her daughter, Mindy, experienced all of the above at a younger age, in addition to emotional and learning differences, autoimmune disease, and chronic pain that made it that much harder to rise to the occasion of her very challenging adolescence and adulthood. And finally, there are Mindy's three children, all born with full mutation fragile X syndrome. At fifteen, Lina can have a sophisticated conversation, though she may bang the table like a toddler if, for example, her opinions about Justin Bieber are challenged. At eighteen, Mike and Aaron need constant supervision.

And Corey: Is he an outlier? Or, as I will argue throughout this book, does his story, and those of other fragile X carriers, model, in all its complexity, the effect of genes on character and fate?

Anyone can see that something is wrong with the twins, Mike and Aaron, boys with fragile X syndrome. That's why the family went to the MIND Institute to get specialty care for them. Many people can see that Lina is atypical, too. But the struggles of the carriers were hidden; if they acknowledged them at all, they blamed themselves or chalked them up to bad luck. Patricia's hoarding, hair-pulling, and the tremulousness that forced her to retire from the bank. Mindy's lifelong anxiety, her dreamlike thought process, her fibromyalgia, her arthritis, her twin pregnancy, her garrulous husband, even the encounter with a coffeepot that left her thigh scarred. Corey, who one day would be shot to death by his own father, with ten hits of methamphetamine tucked away in his fanny pack. What the Solitars learned at the MIND Institute—where they filled out forms and checklists, slid into MRI cylinders, filled vials of blood, and spent hours with researchers in intimate conversation—rewrote the family history. It wasn't just one damn thing after another. It was genes.

Chapter Two

FRAGILE X MUTATIONS

AN OVERVIEW

A SYNDROME is a constellation of physical, intellectual, and emotional *signs*—what doctors see—and *symptoms*—what patients feel. Physically, boys with full mutation fragile X syndrome have poor muscle tone, loose joints, and anomalies of their connective tissues. They tend to have large protruding ears, crowded teeth, and long, narrow faces. Their fingertips may be wide and flat, their feet are flat, their shoulders droop, and their chests cave in. Thanks to their lax connective tissues, they may have remarkably soft, velvety skin and prolapsing heart valves. They are prone to ear infections, gastric reflux, and loose stools. Girls with fragile X syndrome share many of these features, though they are usually less severe. Nearly all fragile X men have large testes—in medical terminology, macroorchidism—which becomes obvious during puberty.

Fragile X syndrome is the most common single-gene form of autism and intellectual disability. Intellectually, most boys with fragile X syndrome have moderate intellectual disability, defined as an IQ in the 35–55 range. Nearly all boys have some features of autism. About one-third of girls with fragile X have mild to moderate intellectual deficits. Some girls are much less affected, with borderline to no intellectual disability, but often have specific learning disabilities and anxiety.[1]

Fragile X syndrome—the full mutation—occurs when an inherited mutation causes the *absence* of a protein called the fragile X mental retardation protein, or FMRP (although the term "mental retardation" has been supplanted by "intellectual disability," the name for the protein remains). Individuals without FMRP or much too little FMRP have fragile X syndrome.

The gene in which the fragile X syndrome mutation occurs has many functions in its normal state. The gene, known as *FMR1*, was identified and sequenced in 1991. The *FMR1* gene provides the instructions for the production of FMRP—the fragile X mental retardation protein. The *FMR1* gene is believed to act as a controller—a powerful gene that manages the expression of many other genes in response to environmental events through its production of FMRP.[2] FMRP is an important protein that functions in the typical brain and helps with communication between different parts of the brain. The shortage of this essential protein causes the deficits seen in fragile X syndrome. Low protein levels inhibit the brain's capacity to respond properly to the outside world.

It is commonly understood that in the duality of nature and nurture, nature means genes. Nurture is harder to define, as it is often assumed to be a synonym for parenting. But nurture really refers to all the experiences that shape us after we are born, even trivial ones. FMRP, which links the brain and the outside world by controlling gene expression, is the *molecular* face of nurture.[3]

GENETICS: A *VERY* QUICK SKETCH

Even the godless science of genetics has a creation myth.[4] A quick sketch of the basics begins with Gregor Mendel, an isolated, unprepossessing Czech monk whose hobby was crossing strains of sweet peas in the monastery garden. Throughout the mid-nineteenth century, by examining how different characteristics such as seed color and stem height sorted over generations, Mendel deduced the basic laws of genetics. These included the idea that traits like stem height and seed color are inherited independently from one another, and that some traits are dominant and some recessive (recessive traits showed up in offspring only when both parents carried the trait). He hypothesized that a unit of information—which would later be named a "gene"— was responsible for carrying these traits from one generation to the next.

Schoolchildren know Gregor Mendel as the "father" of modern genetics. Though its veracity has been doubted, the story goes that Mendel's findings were neglected until 1900—after all, he was an isolated Czech monk—when the Cambridge naturalist William Bateson read his paper "Experiments on Plant Hybridization" aboard that nineteenth-century icon of progress, a moving train. Bateson was on his way to give a lecture, and after reading the paper he changed his talk to introduce his audience to "Mendelism." Bateson's advocacy brought Mendelism into the mainstream.

Meanwhile, in New York City beginning in 1908, Thomas Hunt Morgan and his students at Columbia University's legendary "Fly Lab" were conducting crosses with *Drosophila*, or fruit flies. Fruit flies breed fast, with a new generation every two weeks. Crucially, their traits could be shown to map to large chromosomes, which could be seen with a microscope and photographed. In 1915, Morgan published *The Mechanism of Mendelian Heredity*, the basic text of modern genetics. No longer considered an "ism," Mendel's hypotheses were now established facts.

Though it took some years to get the number right, in the end humans were found to have forty-six chromosomes, two of which are the sex chromosomes, X and Y. Chromosomes were determined to be clumps of genes folded together into a lumpy mass.

In 1944, Oswald Avery's lab in New York identified deoxyribonucleic acid—DNA—as the substance of which genes were made.

In 1953, James Watson and Francis Crick famously demonstrated the double-helix structure of DNA and its implications for how chromosomes and genes replicate themselves. Crick and others went on to show how DNA messages were constructed of four different *bases*—adenine, guanine, cytosine, and thymine. The arrangement of bases in a gene functions as a code; combinations of the four bases tell the cell how to make the different proteins it needs. Genes—made of DNA—form a template, from which many copies of a different molecule called RNA can be made in a process called *transcription*. Through transcription, the DNA message is copied and magnified to make it accessible for a different process, the way a piece of music written for clarinet can be transcribed to be played by a violin. In a subsequent process, called *translation*, the message is transformed further, from genetic code to *protein*. Now, it isn't music at all, but a solid building block—an instrument, say, that with other instruments forms an orchestra. Thus, RNA directs the formation of proteins, which determine the fate of our cells.

This orderly sequence—DNA to RNA to protein—is so well established that it was nicknamed "the central dogma" by James Watson in 1965.

By the mid-1980s, work was underway to map the human genome, which was formalized in 1990 as the Human Genome Project, completed with much self-congratulation in 2003.[5] All that information now lies before us like a buffet from which we can help ourselves.

WOMEN INCLUDED

What this technophilic history neglects is women's work. Years before Bateson read "Experiments on Plant Hybridization" in 1900, he and his wife, Beatrice, experimented with flowers and chickens at home, assisted by college girls who went on to become early geneticists. The young women who attended Cambridge at that time could not obtain degrees, and men grabbed the secure, prestigious academic positions that were available to them, leaving the nascent, then low-status field of genetics free for women.

William Bateson's country compound was a classic example of a premodern laboratory setup for the study of genetics. With a garden, an orchard, outhouses, and animal pens, he and his wife, as historian of science Marsha Richmond writes, "raised chickens, sweet peas, and three sons,"[6] assisted by female students who became part of the household. The women of Girton and Newnham Colleges, the women's colleges of Cambridge University in England, welcomed new opportunities for women to get an education and work in the sciences, and they were drawn to Bateson, whose views on "the woman question" favored their full participation.[7] It was not until a decade or two later, when genetics was better funded and had moved indoors to places like Columbia's Fly Lab, that women became less visible in the new science. They were there, at Columbia and elsewhere, but often acted as lower-paid "assistants" or "administrators" rather than being acknowledged as full-fledged scientists themselves.[8]

The contributions of women to genetics have been strangely overlooked, most infamously in the case of Rosalind Franklin, a codiscoverer of the double helix who was discredited and insulted by James Watson in the most misogynistic terms, with scathing remarks about her looks and personality rather than acknowledgment of her essential scientific contribution.[9]

Nevertheless, women's work is particularly relevant to fragile X disorders. In 1905, Nettie Stevens discovered that male fruit flies had a set of unmatched chromosomes that likely determined their sex.[10] In 1961, Mary Lyon published her findings on "random X-inactivation," which explained why women, with two X chromosomes (men have one X and one Y), don't have a double dose of X-linked genes.[11] One of the X chromosomes is turned off randomly in each cell very early in embryonic development, with significant implications for women with fragile X mutations. Lyon's work showed that in laboratory mice, the gene for coat color was on the X chromosome. Male mice might be one color or another, but female mice could have a random mixture of colors. You can also see this pattern in cats. A male cat might be largely black or orange. But a female cat can have orange and black blended together randomly, in a pattern known as tortoiseshell. The tortoiseshell coloring reflects what is happening—the X-linked genes for hair color are expressed randomly, depending on which X chromosome is turned off in which cell. All tortoiseshell cats are female.

For women with the full mutation, this finding is particularly important. Having more mutated Xs than healthy Xs expressed can make the difference between intellectual disability and normal IQ.

JULIA BELL'S TREASURE

Julia Bell (figure 2.1) first characterized fragile X syndrome. Unable to obtain a mathematics degree from Cambridge in 1901 because of her sex, she went on to become one of the most important figures in the new science of genetics. She was one of a crop of "steamboat ladies"—women who studied at Girton College, Cambridge University's college for women, but were denied degrees from Cambridge. The young men of Cambridge were violently opposed to full admission of women to the university; during an anti-coed protest, they actually burned in effigy a figure of a female student on a bicycle.[12] Fortunately for the young ladies, Trinity College in Ireland was willing to grant degrees to the graduates of Girton, but they had to travel, by steamboat— thus their sobriquet—to Dublin to pick them up in person.

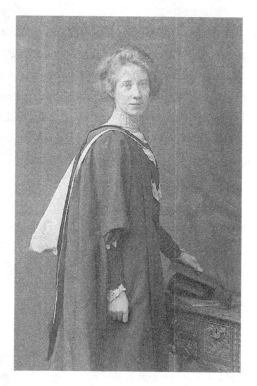

FIGURE 2.1 Julia Bell, then twenty-eight, in her graduation robe, 1907. Originally published in Sarah Bundey, "Julia Bell MRCS LRCP FRCP (1879–1979): Steamboat Lady, Statistician and Geneticist," *Journal of Medical Biography* 4, no. 1 (February 1996): 9.

By 1907, Julia Bell had earned both bachelor's and master's degrees in mathematics at Girton College and steamed to Dublin to obtain her degrees. Geneticist Karl Pearson then hired her as a statistical assistant. She spoke enthusiastically about the "beauty and interest" of statistics, which she said gave her "hopes for the future."[13]

For her planned work on the forthcoming *Treasury of Human Inheritance*, a massive, ever-growing reference book on inherited anomalies, Pearson suggested that she obtain a medical degree. She did so, and now a medical doctor in addition to being a mathematician, she had an impact on medical genetics that might have made her a more familiar name had she been a man.

Bell came of age just as middle-class women were gaining access to universities. She was one of fourteen children, loved literature, and could wield a statistic with empathy. She was drawn to familial conditions, which she described tenderly. And she could count: consanguineous marriages, multiple births, extra fingers. No one had ever attempted to obtain these data before, but it was of tremendous value for medicine to know how many marriages there were between blood relatives, how many triplets had been born that year in England, how many babies had more than ten fingers, and so on. She read widely, found cases in archives, traveled, and took pictures. Her *Treasury of Human Inheritance* was the capstone of a life spent looking, visiting, and counting.

Impediments to obtaining a good family history have been described as "the 6Ds: discernment, distance, divorce, death, denial, and deception."[14] It is clear from Bell's writing that for her these were hardly impediments, but were instead diversions and challenges that made her work all the more fascinating.

The Treasury was remarkable for its collection of inherited diseases and family trees, which it presented without arguing for a particular mechanism, thus avoiding debates over the value of Mendelism. *The Treasury* did not claim to explain how genetic disease was transmitted; it presented evidence and let the informed reader draw his or her own conclusions. Though edited by—and credited to—Karl Pearson and several subsequent heads of Britain's Galton Laboratory between 1909 and 1958, Julia Bell wrote most of it—a true life's work.[15] A 1912 review of an early volume on dwarfism gives a sense of its contents and scope:

> This elaborate volume from the Francis Galton Laboratory for National Eugenics contains a study of the various forms of dwarfism—ethnic dwarfs, achondroplasiacs, the dwarfism of rickets, myxedema, cretinism, and ateliosis or true dwarfism. The subject is treated from all points, including the historical, and a long list of paintings of dwarfs by famous painters is given. The pedigrees of all reported cases, together with eight graphic plates of pedigrees and thirty-five plates of photograph and x-ray illustrations are given of the various classes of dwarfs.[16]

The volume was more than six hundred pages long, exclusive of illustrations.

Bell was a wonderful writer, quoting extensively from great literature and describing the ailing with lively detail. Bell's

"Plural Births with a New Pedigree" is a long literary review and a compendium of bizarre and unbelievable cases of multiple births. She concludes in defense of some of these fantastical cases: "How very incurious most of us appear to be with regard to remarkable occurrences which do not touch upon our own immediate needs and occupations."[17]

Bell and a collaborator, J.B.S. Haldane, were the first scientists to describe the phenomenon of X-linkage in humans (Thomas Hunt Morgan's lab at Columbia University had shown it to exist in flies). They studied families in which hemophilia, a bleeding disorder, and colorblindness were inherited together. Because they so often co-occurred, the genes causing hemophilia and colorblindness had to be located near each other on the same chromosome. And by statistical analysis of the pedigrees of families in which they co-occurred, Bell and Haldane could see that the conditions were passed from mothers who appeared healthy to sons who became ill. That could only be understood if both genes were linked to the X chromosome.

Bell was a remarkable statistician, but she was also a sensitive physician who took an uncommon interest in her patients and their quirks. When an intelligent young mother brought her slow toddler son to Bell's London clinic, concerned that the boy would be an "imbecile" like the sons of her sisters, Bell investigated. Her methods for gathering data were as low-tech as Mendel's scrutiny of seeds. She and a collaborator, J. Purdon Martin, created the child's family tree by examining and interviewing members of many generations and branches, some of whom were not aware of the others or disliked the others so much they made up lies about them. Martin and Bell's 1943 paper "A Pedigree of Mental Defect Showing Sex Linkage" used careful observation and inference to detect a family pattern and described the features of fragile X syndrome that are familiar to clinicians today.[18] The condition came to be known as "Martin-Bell syndrome."

Of three brothers, Bell wrote, "They can answer very simple questions by yes or no; they can say their own names (not always correctly) and the names of the most common objects; none of them can make a sentence. . . . [One], when asked what work he did (carrying coal) after long hesitation and obvious agitation uttered the single word 'black.' "

One was "unemployable, wet, and dirty." Another "hoards rubbish." The fact that the boys' mothers were intellectually normal argued strongly for X-linkage, but some aspects of the pedigree didn't quite fit. Some girls seemed partly affected. One worked as a waitress and could "carry round trays" but could not make change. Another was unable to do arithmetic or work at all outside the home, but she managed to marry "a man of mental equipment similar to her own." There was also a perplexing coda—the inheritance pattern suggested the inexplicable possibility of male carriers. (X-linkage will be discussed further later.) Bell concluded, "The interpretation of this family history from the genetic standpoint is not quite straightforward."

THE COMPLEX WORLD OF FRAGILE X GENETICS

Every disease has its own narrative. When it was first discovered, the fragile X mutation was found to be highly unusual.

Fragile X earned its name because the mutation is found on the X chromosome. Photographed under a microscope and displayed in a karyotype, the X chromosome literally looks like an "X." There is a thin spot near the end of one of the arms of the X, called a fragile site. It looks like a little piece is about to fall off.

Mutations on the X chromosome are known as X-linked mutations. What makes them special is related to the way the X and Y chromosomes dictate whether a baby is a boy or a girl. With very few exceptions, if a baby has two X chromosomes, it is a girl. Again with very few exceptions, if a baby has one X and one Y chromosome, it is a boy.

What this means for X-linked mutations is that they are much more consequential in boys. Because girls nearly always have a healthy X in addition to the X that has a mutation, their healthy X-linked gene compensates for the mutated gene. Boys, on the other hand, have only one X chromosome—the other is a Y. If there is a defect on a boy's X chromosome, there is no other X chromosome to make up for it.

It is helpful to compare fragile X mutations to a better-known, more typical X-linked disease, hemophilia, which killed off the sons of the Russian Empire while leaving their mothers unscathed.[19] Because of a mutation on the X chromosome, people with hemophilia have a defect in a protein, factor VIII, which is necessary for blood to clot. Without factor VIII, affected individuals can bleed profusely from minor injuries. A mother with a mutated factor VIII gene can pass the mutation to her sons, who may die of untreated hemophilia. But the mother herself stays well. Her other X chromosome—the one with no mutation—allows her to produce all the factor VIII she needs.

Mothers like the Russian empresses are *carriers* of an X-linked disease. They don't develop hemophilia, but they pass the condition to their sons, carrying hemophilia to the next generation.

Hemophilia, an X-linked recessive disease, follows Mendel's laws of inheritance. Mendel's laws of dominant and recessive traits imply that carriers of recessive diseases should never have symptoms. A woman with two X chromosomes may have one with a mutation, but the mutated X remains *hidden* behind the healthy one. That is what it means to have a recessive condition. It follows that females may never be diagnosed with recessive diseases on the X chromosome. Their genotypes, their DNA, are different from those of noncarriers, but a carrier's phenotype—how she looks and feels—should be exactly like everyone else's. That is the very definition of being a carrier of a *recessive* Mendelian disorder.

It is now known that fragile X syndrome is different, because it is inherited as an *X-linked dominant disorder.* That means that in women, the unhealthy, mutated X *dominates* over the healthy one, leading to symptoms of disease.

But before the fragile X gene was identified, its inheritance was seen as even more bizarre. It didn't seem to follow the general rules of X-linked inheritance, dominant *or* recessive. For example, men, with only one X chromosome, could be unaffected carriers. And the ratio of affected to unaffected children, which is helpful to geneticists in understanding the mechanism of inheritance, did not make sense.

What the central dogma overlooked was that parts of the gene that did not code for proteins could *also* be significant in health and disease.

Fragile X disorders provide iconic examples of the importance of *epigenetic* changes to DNA that were not appreciated when the central dogma was conceived. The dogma implies that flawed proteins, masterminded by flawed RNA copied from flawed DNA, cause disease. But in fragile X syndrome, FMRP, the protein, is not "flawed." The fragile X mutation lies outside of the protein-coding part of the gene. The mutation triggers chemical modifications to the DNA, termed epigenetic changes, that lead to gene silencing. Because of the mutation, *FMR1* has been turned off, and there just isn't any FMRP at all.[20]

Like other genes, *FMR1* is loaded with repetitive sequences at the front end of the gene. The repetitive sequences in the fragile X gene consist of recurring DNA triplets called *CGG repeats*—threesomes of the bases cytosine and guanine that repeat many times in a burst. It is normal to have CGG repeats—everyone has them in their *FMR1* genes, and everyone has an *FMR1* gene, regardless of their fragile X status. Most people have around thirty CGG repeats in their *FMR1* genes.[21]

People with full mutation fragile X syndrome each have *hundreds* of CGG repeats in the front part of their *FMR1* genes. And when an individual has more than two hundred repeats, many methyl groups—tiny clutches of atoms—get attached to the front part of the gene, the part that regulates its ability to be transcribed. The outcome: the gene is turned off. That is known as an epigenetic modification: a change in gene *expression* that does not alter the genetic code itself and thus does not alter the structure of the protein expressed by the gene.[22]

The CGG expansion is in a *noncoding* part of the gene called the promoter region. The promoter region of a gene does not code for a protein; rather, it is the site that regulates the expression (or transcription) of that gene. In the *FMR1* gene, when the number of CGG repeats reaches greater than 200, the DNA undergoes an epigenetic change. It is *methylated*, rendering the gene silent. The protein needed for normal brain development, FMRP, never gets made. Without FMRP, the individual has symptoms and signs of fragile X syndrome.

This book is called *The Carriers*, and its focus is not on people with fragile X syndrome but on their mothers and fathers and other people who were once considered unaffected by fragile X mutations. It was not understood, until 1991, that large expansions of the CGG repeat cause fragile X syndrome. A small repeat expansion makes the individual a carrier. A much larger expansion, which can only occur in the offspring of people who are carriers, causes fragile X syndrome.

A *carrier* mutation is also known as a *premutation*. Before the fragile X mutation was completely understood, the "pre" referred to the earlier form of the mutation that was not related to symptoms of fragile X syndrome itself, but could *lead* to a full mutation. The way this works is that once the repeat region of the *FMR1* gene has become *unstable* (the initial, or "pre" mutation), it can change in size in each subsequent generation. Most often it begins to expand in size, particularly when passed down from the mother to her child. Eventually, it can expand to a *full* mutation. When the number of CGG repeats reaches or exceeds 200, the full mutation is present.

This will be explained further, but in general in this book, the word "carrier" refers to carriers of a *premutation*. While healthy people have fewer than forty-five CGG repeats, and those with more than two hundred repeats have fragile X syndrome, men and women with a premutation have 55–199 repeats. Those with 45–54 repeats are in the "gray zone," which will also be discussed later. Premutation carriers have two major concerns: health conditions specific to premutation carriers, which are discussed at length in upcoming chapters, and the expansion of their premutation to a full mutation in their children. In other words, premutation carrier women can become mothers of full mutation kids.

OVOIDS AND POLAROIDS

Before a problem can be understood, someone has to notice it, there has to be a language to describe it, and the right people have to investigate it.

Early medical interest in mental retardation was initiated by a Swiss physician, Johann Jakob Guggenbühl, in the mid-nineteenth century. He believed that fresh air, high altitude, and good food, coupled with training, could cure mental retardation. Doctors from all over the world visited his facility and attempted to re-create it in their own countries.[23]

Widely recognized causes of mental retardation at that time included syphilis, cretinism (caused by low iodine), and Down syndrome, a particular problem back then as women continued having children until menopause, and Down syndrome is associated with advanced maternal age. Consanguinity—unions between blood relatives—was another frequent cause of intellectual and other disabilities and was said to decrease when the bicycle was invented and people could travel to more distant gene pools.

In the United States, the 1890 census reported a male preponderance of the "feeble-minded or idiotic" in institutions, without comment.[24] The term "genetics," coined by Bateson, first appeared in 1905.[25]

Eugenicists of the early twentieth century promoted the idea that certain unfortunate families were destined by genes to bring more mentally retarded individuals into the world, including some families that became household names through tabloids and books. For the most part, though, the idea of "cultural familial retardation" predominated during the first half of the twentieth century. This was a wastebasket term that applied to mental retardation of any type without an obvious cause. Meanwhile, as clinical psychologist Robert Gordon Lehrke writes, the "excess of male retardates appears to have been accepted as one of the facts of life, like gravity, the weather, or taxes."[26]

A significant and sorry development in the history of intellectual disability was the warehousing of the intellectually disabled into institutions throughout the early twentieth century. This had the effect of isolating not only the disabled but also their caregivers and the professionals who took an interest in them. It is no coincidence that research in intellectual disability began to snowball as these institutions were closed in the late 1950s and early 1960s.

This new wave of medical interest in intellectual disability began in 1956, the year that the human chromosomes were first clearly seen and counted. The study of chromosomes as they pertain to heredity is known as *cytogenetics*, and for geneticists, this period became known as the "cytogenetic era."

An extra chromosome—a third copy of chromosome 21, or trisomy 21—was discovered to be the cause of Down syndrome in 1958. Most of the trisomies (third copies) and partial deletions (missing bits of genetic information) were described by 1960. Major hospitals opened cytogenetics departments in the early 1960s. Around this time, a deeper understanding grew concerning inborn errors of metabolism—in which waste products build up and destroy the central nervous system and other organs—such as Tay-Sachs disease and phenylketonuria (PKU). Pediatricians and geneticists were suddenly more interested in children with intellectual disability, which now could be prevented by a special diet in the case of PKU or by selective abortion in the case of Tay-Sachs, and they started to look for patterns of minor external features of physical abnormality.

A serendipitous boost was the invention of the Polaroid camera, which allowed doctors to photograph patients' faces on the spot and slip a picture into their files, making it easier to recognize recurring features in different disorders.[27]

The range of normal measurements for a variety of physical features was documented. In 1966, an endocrinologist, Dr. Andrea Prader, standardized the expected volume of the testes by age, so pediatricians had a norm by which to measure a boy's development.

Testicular size was difficult to measure. Basically a pediatrician would grab a wriggling boy's testis and guess its volume. Prader invented the orchidometer, which was a circle of beads on a string with ovoids of different volumes.[28] A doctor could hold a patient's testis in one hand and feel for the same-size "testis" on the orchidometer with the other. Thus, testicular size could be estimated more accurately, which later helped identify the enlargement of the testes in fragile X syndrome.

In 1969, Herbert Lubs reported on a "marker X" chromosome in the affected males of a family with Martin-Bell syndrome. A constriction at the end of one of the arms of the X, the marker was a fragile site that appeared to pinch the chromosome, so that it looked like a little piece could break off at any time. The discovery of the fragile site was an important finding in research into Martin-Bell syndrome. When an individual from a Martin-Bell family was symptomatic, he had a fragile site on his X chromosome. An individual from the same family, but without intellectual impairment, had no fragile site. Lubs further found an association between the fragile site and enlarged testes, or macroorchidism.[29]

In a 1983 reminiscence, Australian geneticist Gillian Turner wrote, "Having something that one can count or measure, that is always present in the presence of disease and never present in the absence of disease, is an enormous step forward. This is why the discovery of the fragile site is so important."[30] The same could be said of the orchidometer, which allowed macroorchidism to be characterized as either present or absent.

NOT QUITE STRAIGHTFORWARD

Throughout the early 1970s, and culminating with the publication of his thesis, "X-linked Mental Retardation and Verbal Disability," Robert Gordon Lehrke labored over the issue of X-linked mental retardation. For reasons still unclear to me, the idea of an increased incidence of intellectual disability in males was met with skepticism, even outrage. Institutional records clearly showed that males were overrepresented, but data on intellectual disability from institutional records was thought to be an artifact of institutionalization. There was a sense that males caused more trouble in the community, and there were higher expectations for them if they were to function in the general population; thus, they were more likely to be institutionalized. In contrast, there may have been more tolerance for intellectually disabled girls in the community, though some girls may have been institutionalized to prevent pregnancy. However, by the late 1950s, it had been shown that institutional populations accurately reflected community populations. Lehrke proposed that it was a simple fact that males are overrepresented in intellectually disabled populations and put forth an elegant argument on why X-linked mental retardation (XLMR) was the reason.

Lehrke's theory of XLMR included four hypotheses:

1. There are genes on the X chromosome relating to intellectual function.
2. These genes if mutated lead to mental retardation transmitted in an X-linked manner.

3. One or more genes relates to verbal function (differentiated from global function).

4. The deficit relates to the central nervous system (i.e., not the entire body).

Lehrke's work used statistical analysis to argue that all of these hypotheses were true.[31]

Why had no one noticed X-linked mental retardation before? Lehrke highlighted social factors: "Staffs of schools [and] social work agencies . . . lack persons with the knowledge of genetics that would make appropriate pedigree analysis possible."[32] It would take the founding of academic medical centers such as the MIND Institute to gather these professionals together. He further suggested that a "highly mobile society leaves us at a disadvantage. It is rare that large families over several generations remain in the same community."[33]

Another source of confusion, he guessed, was that the overall functioning of individuals with XLMR would depend as well upon other genetic and environmental factors. These other factors, which apply more nearly equally to both sexes, would conceal the pattern of X-linkage in most families. Another concealing factor is the presence—especially relevant for fragile X syndrome—of mildly affected girls.[34]

Lehrke hypothesized that 20–36 percent of mental retardation is associated with X-linked genes. He called this excess of males over females "an army of male retardates,"[35] an upsetting term to hear today.

"Martin-Bell syndrome" was the first form of X-linked intellectual disability ever described; we now recognize more than two hundred of them.[36] In the early 1980s, geneticists located surviving members of the original family described by Martin and Bell. DNA tests showed that they carried a mutation on the X chromosome at the so-called fragile site. The identity of Martin-Bell syndrome and fragile X syndrome was established, and the name fragile X syndrome replaced Martin-Bell.[37]

■ ■ ■

In 1986, researcher John M. Opitz gave a talk at one of the first international conferences centered on X-linked mental retardation. In addition to thanking Robert Lehrke (not coincidentally, his thesis advisee), Opitz commented that fragile X syndrome was "not a conventional Mendelian condition."[38]

Fourteen years later, in 2000, Opitz gave a historical address. He said, in an echo of Bateson's dynamic "rediscovery" of Mendel on his way to an academic lecture:

Everything (almost everything) became suddenly clear in the spring of 1991 when three independent groups . . . came up with the gene of the fragile X syndrome, *FMR1*, and with the brand-new concept of instability of a triplet (CGG) repeat as a mutational mechanism causing anticipation and distortion of the classic mendelian pattern of inheritance. More than that, *FMR1* turned out to be only the first example of an ever-growing class of such dynamic mutations. One personal (G.N.) recollection of that exhilarating moment is that of rushing to a genetics meeting in Southern Italy, holding a hardly legible and incomplete telefax copy of the Verkerk paper, and announcing to a puzzled audience that yes, human genes can also mutate by just becoming bigger than they normally are.[39]

To paraphrase, yes, human genes can mutate by expansion of CGG repeat length, enlarging the gene. Eureka!

Chapter Three

VILLAGE OF FOOLS

HOW CARRIERS BROUGHT FRAGILE X TO COLOMBIA, AND WHAT HAPPENED NEXT

RICAURTE IS a village in Colombia, about seventy-five miles northeast of Cali in the Valle del Cauca, a wide plain planted with sugarcane between two strands of the Andes. It has the highest concentration of individuals with fragile X mutations in the world. Its isolation and the intellectual disability of its population led to tragic consequences during Colombia's decades-long civil conflict, particularly since the 1980s, and as a result of the proximity of the cocaine trade. Ricaurte's men were easily led on by thugs and then shot to death, their bodies left to present a show of might to enemies. Many of Ricaurte's women were alleged to have been attacked and raped. It was rumored that these rapes led to the birth of more babies with intellectual disability.[1]

Local folks who knew of Ricaurte were aware of its remarkable population of "*bobitos*," or "fools." The *bobitos* earned a few coins watching the parked cars of pilgrims who visited the village's holy site, where *El Divino Ecce Homo*, a painting said to grant miracles, was enshrined in a plain church.[2]

I had been studying fragile X mutations for several years and had become intrigued with this little village of misfortune. It was a long-held dream for me to travel there and see it with my own eyes. There were two things I hoped to learn by traveling to Ricaurte. First, how did this tiny, off-the-map village become the planet's densest hotspot for fragile X? What could it teach me about fragile X population genetics? And second, given its remoteness and its lack of access to many of the twenty-first century's modern amenities, how did scientists all over the world come to know about it? What could Ricaurte show me about scientific progress?

SCIENCE AND SORCERY

Ricaurte's intellectually disabled men and women once struggled daily with aggression, victimization, and shame. Many were unable to have a meaningful conversation, most had autistic features, and some had no words at all. They were typically lanky, with large ears, light blue eyes, floppy flat feet, and a tendency to avoid eye contact. Some, especially the men, were always active, while others, especially the women, were in wheelchairs or would only move when led by the hand.

During the 1980s, a prominent Colombian author and local politician, Gustavo Alvarez Gardeazabal, wrote *El divino*, a novel set in the village, and in 1988 a soap opera based on the book was wildly popular on television.[3] Rumors about the

village and its mysterious maladies swirled. Villagers and out-
siders as well had several theories.

One was that its men had been poisoned by *chamico*, or jimson weed, used by Ricaurte's women in a form of witchcraft
intended to make men fall in love with them. Young men were
warned never to drink anything given to them by a woman in
Ricaurte.

Less colorful hypotheses for the high rate of intellectual disability included the concentration of magnesium that flowed
through the nearby Cauca River, marriage between relatives,
and the idea that "bad families" brought intellectual disability
to Ricaurte. In the end, the last was closest to the truth.[4]

Nothing livens things up like a good story. We tend to
think of doctors as staid, fact-oriented individuals, but good
stories come in many forms and may appear as unusual case
reports in the peer-reviewed journals that doctors subscribe
to. On occasion—as I did—we might open a journal and with
a little imagination find ourselves immersed in a spectacu-
lar lurid tale featuring sexually starved women wielding
aphrodisiacs.

Tabloid fodder, like sorcery, is a type of medical technology:
perhaps not necessary, but surely sufficient, to bring a new diagnosis to medical attention. Early on, a bizarre medical detail
catches a young person's eye. Later, once immersed in the topic,
it captures his or her mind, and finally, heart. No one illustrates
this sequence better than Wilmar Saldarriaga Gil, a medical
geneticist and gynecologist in Cali.

Wilmar, forty-five at the time of this writing, grew up spending summers visiting his grandfather in Ricaurte's neighboring

village of Huasano. His investigation of Ricaurte began as a boy's fascination with unusual people—*bobitos* whom he saw in town at church. As a young medical student in the mid- to late 1990s, his intellectual interest continued. He paged through an enormous textbook filled with photographs of people with congenital anomalies. He found pictures of patients with long faces, big ears, floppy limbs, and intellectual and particularly marked verbal disabilities. The patients in the photographs had fragile X syndrome. Wilmar was struck by the similarities between what he saw in the textbook and the men and women of Ricaurte. He wanted to meet the residents, and he wanted to take samples of their blood to look for the telltale mutation. Because of his personal history and interests, he was the first person to find a plausible scientific explanation for this peculiar population.

Wilmar began traveling to the village on a regular basis, his natural friendliness, insider status, and calm demeanor making him a welcome visitor. He visited hundreds of homes, nearly all of the village's population of 1,300 or so residents. He took a detailed history from the eldest member of each household, inquiring about everything they could remember about their parents and grandparents and other family lore. He used local historical documents and land deeds to establish the connections between today's residents of Ricaurte and its founders. In-depth personal interviews were essential because of the large number of extramarital unions that could have created confusion in the lineages of the different families.[5]

Eventually Wilmar's evident trustworthiness and genuine concern for the welfare of the population of Ricaurte persuaded those whom he believed fit the fragile X profile to give him blood samples, allowing him to trace their genealogy. He used the best technology available to him at the time, which allowed him to prepare a karyotype, or photograph, of an individual's chromosomes. The test results showed the telltale sign: a tiny notch near one end of the X chromosome. Wilmar was right: Ricaurte's *bobitos* had fragile X syndrome.

THE FOUNDERS

The settlement of Ricaurte began around the beginning of the nineteenth century. The village was something of a planned community whose original name was Yeguerizo, an area for breeding livestock. Eleven families converged from different parts of Colombia to develop the village.[6] Colombia's genetic ancestral background is a mixture of Indigenous, Spanish, and African DNA. According to documents about the founding of Ricaurte, the families of some of the founders came directly from Spain.

Matching lab results to the extensive multigenerational pedigree Wilmar's door-to-door interviews had produced, Wilmar could see that most of the families who had fragile X disorders had Spanish surnames; in fact, many were the surnames of some of the village's founders.[7] By inference, he hypothesized that one to four particular families brought fragile X to Ricaurte. Each of today's full mutation or premutation carriers in Ricaurte is descended from one of these families. This is known as a *founder effect*.

In a founder effect, a single family (or a small group of people) brings a genetic mutation to an isolated area, often an island or a faraway place like Ricaurte. Here, because of the remoteness of the village, surrounded by mountains, few people could come and go. The mutation established itself, not through poisoned water or witchery but through, as one rumor had it, "bad families"—more properly, through families with mutated genes. These families had happened to carry the mutation along unknowingly when Ricaurte was established two centuries ago.

Wilmar believes that the carriers were probably the colonists from Spain.[8] They brought fragile X to Ricaurte, where their daughters inherited their fathers' X chromosomes, becoming carriers themselves. The carriers may have had no symptoms. As the generations descended, the prevalence of the full syndrome and the carrier state increased to an astonishing percentage of the citizenry. A 1999 study of Ricaurte showed that thirty-five individuals had full mutation fragile X syndrome, out of 1,128 inhabitants.[9] This was more than three hundred times the generally accepted rate of fragile X syndrome in the rest of the world.

EL PUEBLO DE LOS BOBOS

Flying a long distance always feels like magic. In New York, it was 17 degrees, but when I got out of the airport in Cali at 10:00 p.m., a tropical breeze blew the scent of asphalt and jet fuel around the parking lot. Wilmar was waiting in a little cluster of people meeting planes. Wilmar is tall, with very dark hair

and eyes, fair skin, and bee-stung lips. Right away his gracious-
ness was apparent. We got to his house in a gated middle-class
neighborhood in Cali, and I went straight to bed in his ten-year-
old daughter's lovely room with peace-and-love bedding, spar-
kly pillows, and stickers with mottoes like "love" and "good
vibes." I was feeling them.

In the morning we drove northeast to Ricaurte, stopping
along the way to pick up Laura Gonzalez, Wilmar's research
assistant for the past six years. Luckily for me she spoke perfect
English, even suggesting I sit in the "shotgun seat," which I
found both impressive as a feat of fluency and very considerate.

Once we left Cali, the fields were green, though Wilmar
bemoaned sugarcane farming as unfortunate for villagers,
because it requires so few workers and contributes to unemploy-
ment. As the morning went on the temperature outside rose to
over 100 degrees.

Just as Wilmar had been warned away from drinks in
Ricaurte by his father years ago, so had I been warned not to
drink the water outside of major cities. But we stopped in Bolivar, a small town a stone's throw from Ricaurte, for lunch, and
were served limeade from a big glass jug with a polystyrene soup
container floating in it like a little white sailboat on a green sea.
The waiter would reach into the jug and scoop up a soup container of limeade to refill our glasses. I realized that hygienic
warnings, jimson weed, or no, I would be drinking the local
water. In fact, at every house we visited in Ricaurte, women
brought us glasses of fresh juice.

Ricaurte had a welcoming entrance with a paved road and a
proud sign, Yo (♥=amo) Ricaurte, "I love Ricaurte," with letters

in primary colors. Tropical flowers grew here and there, and the houses, made mostly of cement, crumbling bricks, and drywall, were painted in faded pinks, oranges, and greens. Laura remarked that six years ago, when she started coming to Ricaurte, roads were not paved and the place was a lot more run down. Wilmar also said that the village looks better than ever, pointing out a central square with grass and playground equipment that just a few years ago was a patch of dirt, and a health center, staffed for our visit by a nurse and a young doctor in mint green scrubs.

As soon as we got out of the car, we applied sunscreen, put on sunglasses and hats, and sprayed ourselves all over with mosquito repellent. It was dengue season.

We began with a full mutation family that Wilmar suspects is one of the founding families which brought the mutation from Spain at the turn of the eighteenth century.[10] They live near the village entrance. Wilmar asked Laura and me to wait outside because one of the men, Diego, is known to be erratic and always carries a machete.[11] Wilmar would go first as Diego would recognize him. It turned out that Diego wasn't there. We followed Wilmar along a little dirt path to a crumbling home with chickens running about the living room. When Wilmar first came to the village, the family had no electricity or refrigerator, and Wilmar raised the funds to get both installed. He immediately checked the lights and looked in the fridge. The four middle-aged brothers and sisters who live there all have fragile X syndrome—their deceased mother was a carrier—and they let the food go bad sometimes. The only one home at first was a sister, who was mopping the floor. She was very happy to see Wilmar, who gave her a loaf of fresh bread. He weighed her and took measurements of her head, the distance between her eyes, and the "prognathism" of her jaw (her underbite). He posed a few questions, such as whether she could read or write (no) and sign her name (yes), and asked that she show him her Colombian ID card. She answered all his questions unselfconsciously. Then Diego returned with his machete. Inside the house, he careened around, never letting go of the machete. He was not threatening, but he was careless. He was bare-chested. He wanted to show us his garden, which Laura said he does at every visit. He had two rabbits in cages and chickens everywhere. He had large bunches of plantains growing and used his machete skillfully to cut some down and trim them to give to Wilmar.

We next went to the home of an eighty-three-year-old woman who is a premutation carrier. Altagracia is the small, sweet matriarch of a family of three sons with fragile X syndrome, a daughter with both fragile X and Down syndromes, and a daughter who is a premutation carrier, but unusually impaired. Altagracia has no overt disability, in fact, she has thrived over the years while managing a challenging brood of children, some of whom are now in their sixties. We spent quite a bit of time with this family, eating the fresh bread Wilmar had brought and drinking coffee, while Altagracia spoke with Wilmar about her biggest worry: who will care for her children when she is no longer able to do so.

Of the adult men, only one is able to work. He came to the porch with a stick with a rope attached—he is a cattle worker who also breaks horses. Another son, Jorge, hangs around the house and is quite goofy, nonverbal, with one snaggle tooth. Like Wilmar, he was wearing a Vallecaucana University polo shirt. They hugged and posed for a picture.

Wilmar told me that another son, who was not present, is unfortunately into drugs and alcohol and at some points has been sexually abused and humiliated by men in nearby Bolivar in exchange for substances. The day after a binge, he often has prolonged seizures, which further damage his brain. The daughter with both fragile X and Down syndromes, Altagracia's youngest, was doll-like. She had a constant smile on her face, tiny cupped ears, and very dark eyes with epicanthal folds. She did not speak. She is too frail to stand or walk herself; she needs support, perhaps because she has very flat, tiny feet that look like they have no bones. She needed help to stand up from a chair and was led around like a baby.

Finally, there was Altagracia's other daughter, who is in her late fifties and a premutation carrier; she is very severely affected and wheelchair-bound. Like some (rare) carriers, she has a seizure disorder. Because of the limited options available in Ricaurte for anti-epileptic medications, she was treated with phenobarbital, which can cause neurotoxicity. She appears to follow a conversation but doesn't speak. She used to walk as a child but stopped at some point, and no one knows why. Though she has the long face, large ears, and light blue eyes common to those with fragile X syndrome, she has been tested twice and is definitely a premutation carrier.

Wilmar believes that carriers in Ricaurte may have other genetic "hits" that predispose them to more severe symptoms. Taken together, Ricaurte's carriers had the worst symptoms I have ever seen in carriers. Many had autism, seizures, and mood disorders in addition to difficulty walking and tremor. Some were indistinguishable from brothers and sisters with the full mutation, though repeated tests had shown them to be "merely" carriers. For Altagracia's daughter, it seems likely that an unin-tentional overdose of phenobarbital played a role in the onset of her profound disability.[12] She was also one of many residents of Ricaurte who are chronically exposed to organophosphates and other pesticides, which they store in their homes to use in their gardens.

Before we left Altagracia's home, Wilmar took lots of pictures. I was surprised at how relaxed the adults with fragile X syndrome were around us and each other, standing close together to pose. Many men with fragile X recoil from close contact and don't look strangers or even loved ones in the eye. It's too stressful for them. But here, no one seemed uncomfortable. They put their arms around each other, and every member of the family was clearly delighted to be near to Wilmar. "He is a celebrity," whispered Laura. When Wilmar was ill several years ago, the entire village prayed for him, and masses were said in his name.

Wilmar and Laura were eager to check in on Julieta, a younger well woman who is also a premutation carrier. She had a new baby, about four months old. Wilmar explained why this visit was so important to him. When the diagnoses of fragile X syndrome were first made in the village, carriers with the premutation were identified as well. Julieta was one of ten premutation carriers of childbearing age. She was the only one of the ten who had not chosen to be sterilized after genetic counseling.

The other nine women, some of whom already had children, chose sterilization, because so many had brothers with fragile X syndrome, or at least had seen what fragile X had done to many of the inhabitants of Ricaurte.[13]

Julieta's house was dark and in disrepair. She looked exhausted, as many mothers of infants do. Right over her head, above the couch, was an idealized portrait of her graduating from high school, holding a rolled-up diploma. She looked glamorous and hopeful in the picture. Her baby boy nursed vigorously, which was a good sign for him, as a "poor suck" can be a symptom of fragile X syndrome in infants. The grandmother brought out glasses of "tree tomato" juice, which Laura told me was a taste it took years to acquire. I took a few sips, embarrassed by my inability to drink it down. The new mother appeared depressed. Wilmar asked to speak with her alone. He very much wanted to test the baby to see if he had a mutation. She agreed, and we planned to return to draw blood.

A bit later we sat outside the elementary school in the central square and chatted with another premutation carrier mother whose healthy eight-year-old son attends the school. She too looked distracted and sad, but when Wilmar asked her if she had any regrets about being sterilized—seven years ago, *after* her son was born—she brightened, laughed, and said she would have done it sooner if she had known she was a premutation carrier. Given that she had a healthy son, that surprised me. Her desire to avoid having a child with fragile X syndrome was so strong that she would have passed up the chance to have that thriving boy, just to be sure.

THE SHERMAN PARADOX

All mothers of individuals with fragile X syndrome have either a full mutation or a premutation. Women with full mutation fragile X syndrome have a 50 percent chance of passing the mutated X to their children and giving birth to children with fragile X syndrome.

When a female premutation carrier like Julieta has a child, there are three possibilities. She can pass her healthy X chromosome to the child. She can pass an expanded full mutation to her child, who will be born with fragile X syndrome.

Finally, she can pass her premutation to the child, who will also have a premutation—generally, with more CGG repeats than the mother. The premutation is unstable, and the CGG repeat length tends to "grow" with each generation.

For a carrier mother, the more CGG repeats she has, the more likely it is that her premutation will expand to a full mutation. The lower end of the carrier range was established to be 55, because 56 repeats is the lowest number ever observed to expand to a full mutation in one generation. As the number of repeats increases above 55, the odds that it will expand to a full mutation increase as well. For example, a woman with 60 repeats has a low likelihood of passing a full mutation to her child, though it's possible. For a woman with over 100 CGG repeats, the likelihood of full mutation fragile X syndrome in her children is essentially 100 percent if the child inherits the mutated X.[14]

Because the unstable premutation keeps growing, each generation is more likely than the previous to have a child affected with fragile X syndrome. In the case of fragile X, this situation has been dubbed the *Sherman paradox*.[15] The Sherman paradox was named after the population geneticist Stephanie Sherman, who noticed and defined it during an early fragile X conference in 1986. Perhaps paradoxically, it is not a paradox at all but a then-inexplicable phenomenon she discovered: healthy men have more descendants with fragile X than they have brothers with fragile X.

More specifically, this refers to the unusual situation of so-called "normal transmitting males." These are *male* carriers of an X-linked disease (remember that males don't have another X chromosome to help weaken the effect of an X-linked mutation, so in more typical diseases, like hemophilia, they are fully affected), a very rare phenomenon. For reasons still not understood, the premutation expands to a full mutation only when passed from females, not males. Because men pass their X chromosome to daughters only, *none of the sons* of a normal transmitting male get their father's X-linked mutation. But *all of the daughters* of normal transmitting males will be premutation carriers too, and *they* can become mothers of children with fragile X syndrome. The end result: "normal transmitting males" are likely to become ancestors of children with full mutation fragile X syndrome.

The Sherman paradox describes the phenomenon we saw in the Solitar family: Thomas, the great-grandfather, had several siblings, but none with fragile X syndrome. However, all three of his great-grandchildren have it.

In 1991, when the premutation was discovered to be a long string of CGG repeats with the potential to expand with each generation, the so-called paradox was "resolved." Because of this unusual inheritance pattern, the founder effect is only a partial explanation for the exponential rise in cases of fragile X syndrome in Ricaurte. That is, the founders and those older generations carried the *FMR1* premutation, but they never knew it. They didn't have symptoms of fragile X syndrome. They did pass the premutation through many generations, however, and it expanded in size with each generation. The Sherman paradox, along with the founder effect, lies behind the unusual population of carriers and full mutation individuals in tiny Ricaurte.

ON THE MAP

A Colombian American social worker, Sergio Villada, brought Wilmar's years of walking the alleys of Ricaurte collecting blood samples and even more precious family histories to the attention of the international research community.

Familial disease is a wellspring of medical progress. Every medical professional knows that for many, interest in medicine, or often in a particular condition, starts with adjusting to the illnesses of oneself or a family member. While Wilmar was studying medicine in Cali, Sergio Villada was growing up in Broward County, Florida. His immediate family had fled Colombia to avoid its civil war and terror attacks. They were preceded to south Florida by an aunt who came to the United States to get specialized treatment for her son. He had intellectual disability and was not getting his needs met. Sergio's cousin had fragile X syndrome, which doctors in Colombia were not generally aware of. "We learned it was hereditary, and all the family had to be tested. But no one could guide us on the right path," Sergio explained.[16]

In fact, Sergio's family was profoundly affected by fragile X disorders. His mother had two uncles in Colombia who were considered to be "crazy" and spent their lives locked inside. Two cousins, who are carriers, suffer from autism. They are able to live independently, but they have difficulty making decisions and managing unforeseen situations. They need novel ideas to be explained to them several times.

When he was in his mid-twenties, Sergio spent two years back in Colombia with his wife and daughter. That was when he heard about Ricaurte, which he told me was known in English as "the town of the dummies." Some of the stories he heard—whether truth, exaggeration, or myth—were quite shocking: rapes, murders, involuntary sterilization, drug addiction, prostitution. The intellectually disabled citizens of Ricaurte were easily victimized. Sergio felt compelled to raise awareness of the plight of Ricaurte's *bobitos* and of fragile X in Colombia in general. Inevitably his journey led him to Wilmar.

Once he was back home in the United States, Sergio reached out to the National Fragile X Foundation and the MIND Institute of the University of California, Davis. He was looking for funding for a film he wanted to make about fragile X in Colombia. In this way, he became the conduit who brought Wilmar's work to the attention of researchers at the MIND Institute.

The institute's scientists were fascinated by the Colombian cluster of fragile X syndrome. There are several such clusters, in places as far apart as Israel, Finland, and Tunisia. There is also a higher incidence of fragile X in the Spanish province of Extremadura, in southwestern Spain, a poor, landlocked area from which many young men left to become *conquistadores*.

Between Wilmar, Sergio, the National Fragile X Foundation, and the staff at the MIND Institute, the Colombia Project of Hope was born. The Project's first visit to Ricaurte took place in 2013. Its goals included universal testing, more technically advanced testing, genetic counseling, and establishing basic health care in Ricaurte.

EL DIVINO

Late in the afternoon, after our family visits, we went to the cathedral to see Ricaurte's icon, *El Divino*. Wilmar remarked upon the fine condition of the church, the newly repaired pews, and the fresh paint. The church looked as if it had been erected for a fair—an unadorned A-frame, painted white, simple, with a soaring open space, almost like a barn where animals would be shown. This is where the idol, *El Divino*, is kept upstairs in a little altar.

It was surrounded by a silver frame and encased in a glass cabinet. It looked like it had been painted by a very gifted child who had not quite mastered perspective. *El Divino* is a portrait of Jesus, nearly nude, pensive, resting his cheek against one hand, with many wounds and a crown of thorns, who appears to be behind two lengths of barbed wire. Its tragic simplicity seems an appropriate emblem for Ricaurte. Since the Project of

Hope began, there is also a mural representing *El Divino* painted on the side of the school building on the central square (figure 3.1). Around *El Divino* in the mural are pictures of the people with fragile X of Ricaurte, with the faces of the individuals drawn in detail. I recognized several men, including Altagracia's sons—that snaggle tooth!—and her daughter with Down syndrome.

Wilmar seems to take much less credit than he deserves for how life in Ricaurte has improved since he came to understand it medically. He diagnosed fragile X syndrome and the carrier

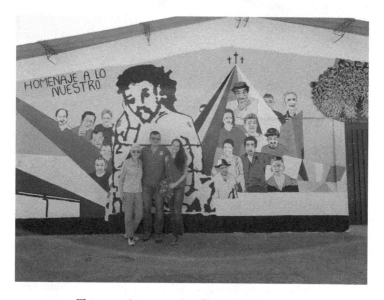

FIGURE 3.1 This mural is painted in Ricaurte's main square. A reproduction of *El Divino* is surrounded by portraits of the citizens of Ricaurte affected by fragile X syndrome. In front of *El Divino*, from left to right: the author, Wilmar Saldarriaga Gil, and Laura Yuriko González Teshima. Photographer unknown, 2020.

state and provided genetic counseling that has so reduced the birth rate of people with fragile X disorders that today there is only one six-year-old with fragile X syndrome from Ricaurte (and perhaps the infant we saw on our visit). Otherwise the inhabitants with fragile X syndrome are mostly much older, in their forties to eighties, and the carriers are too, except for those young women who have been surgically sterilized after learning about the inheritance of fragile X disorders.

Equally significant, his efforts, along with Sergio's and the Project of Hope's, brought basic health care, paved roads, and in some areas, electricity, to Ricaurte. Wilmar now has a twenty-plus-year relationship with the *bobitos*, has paid for and installed their refrigerators, repaired their roofs, drunk their juices, and eaten from their gardens. In return, the *bobitos* have given him a distinguished career and an international reputation.

For the villagers, being given a diagnosis for their mysterious condition did wonders for local pride. Once the town of the *bobitos* had lived in shame. Now they knew who they were. They shine alongside *El Divino* in the center of town.

■ ■ ■

Ricaurte's rescue from abject poverty is an example of the power of "small" science, of door-to-door visits and interviews about private behavior rather than high-tech stuff. Ricaurte's worst problems were not resolved by scientific breakthroughs but through Wilmar's fieldwork and heart. The interventions that came out of the Project of Hope, from the point of view of the villagers' quality of life, had little to do with the precise diagnosis and the sophisticated genetic techniques that made it possible. From the point of view of the researchers at the MIND Institute, the diagnosis was already obvious. Wilmar had found it in a book. The genetic tests were just confirmatory.

Ricaurte has the highest incidence of fragile X syndrome anywhere in the world, thanks to the combination of a founder effect and the unstable CGG repeats in the *FMR1* gene, specifically in the premutation. It came to the attention of the wider scientific community through the efforts of Wilmar, whose curiosity about the area began in childhood, and Sergio, who took it upon himself to bring better medical care to developmentally disabled Colombians like his cousin.

James Watson and Francis Crick, who discovered the structure of DNA, are also known for their maxims: the "boredom principle" and the "gossip test," respectively.[17] Watson advised, "Never do anything that bores you," and Crick said, "What you are really interested in is what you gossip about." Wilmar's work and Sergio's are fine examples of what can happen in science when passion fuses with curiosity.

Chapter Four

A CLASSIC ZEBRA

FRAGILE X–ASSOCIATED PRIMARY OVARIAN INSUFFICIENCY (FXPOI)

ARIEL WAS the youngest of three children, with two big brothers.[1] Her middle brother, James, was diagnosed with fragile X syndrome in 1989, when he was nine years old and she was four. A cousin who happened to be an occupational therapist became concerned about his behavior at a family dinner. Planning her own family, the cousin asked if James could be evaluated for an inherited disorder. Family testing revealed James's full mutation diagnosis, and that Ariel's eldest brother, Franklin, had a normal X chromosome. Ariel was found to have a premutation with about 100 CGG repeats.

With James struggling in a class for kids with learning disabilities, his mother, Belle, was not one to wait around for things to improve. The diagnosis stunned Belle, whose can-do attitude and always positive outlook had led her to minimize James's intellectual disability. "Before, I kept thinking, with a pair of glasses, he'll learn to read."[2] After meeting with the genetic counselor, that fantasy deflated. Her grief, however, lasted less than an hour. "I changed my attitude and embraced it."

James was in a class for kids with learning disabilities and normal to above-normal IQ. "I realized how generous everybody was," Belle now says, to think he had a normal IQ. "I knew nothing about mental retardation or special needs." Belle learned everything she could about James's condition, refused to feel shamed by his diagnosis, and cultivated relationships with anyone she felt could be helpful to James and get him the best education. She knew she couldn't help James by sitting around and complaining.

Ariel may have inherited a premutation from her mother, but she also inherited her mother's grit and optimism. She was an excellent student and a competitive athlete. She won several awards in high school and was named "best all-around student." At sixteen, she turned an English class homework assignment into a ninety-three-page book called *My eXtra Special Brother*,[3] about the joys and challenges of growing up with James. In the book, which is aimed at middle-schoolers, Ariel acknowledged how tough it was to tolerate her brother's sometimes embarrassing displays in public places and how awkward it could be to introduce him to her friends. At the same time she celebrated him for his sense of humor, his guts, and his warmth. The book draws power from its unreserved honesty and the charming illustrations of James and family drawn by a friend of Ariel's. The cover of the book includes photos of James, Ariel, and Franklin and their parents; this is a family that tolerates no shame about James's diagnosis but acknowledges that as she grew up with James, Ariel was not her best self every minute of

every day. I think any sibling of a special needs child would recognize herself in it. Ariel was able to write it because she was
open-hearted, patient, forthright, and ambitious.

That's why it was so startling when Ariel's state of mind
began to change as high school drew to a close. It started with
hot flashes and night sweats. Over a few months Ariel's parents added three vents to her ceiling to cool her room down.
She was moody, anxious, and increasingly depressed. She had
gotten into her first-choice college, and, as she says, "Usually I
thrive off transitions." But she began to dread leaving home. She
was jittery and couldn't concentrate, and her weight dropped.
She did make it to college, but she lasted only a few weeks. At
a low point she called her mother and told her she could see how
a person might consider suicide.

Belle did not take that lightly, and she drove Ariel home and
straight to a psychiatrist. "The next three years was a big fog,"
Ariel told me. She spent all her time in her room, never answered
the phone, and passed the time listening to Enya, the Irish
singer-songwriter whose videos of rain falling on wet leaves
captivate the depressed. She went back and forth between psychiatrists and medical doctors looking for the root of her problem. Visits to the doctor showed abnormal levels of several
hormones some of the time, but sometimes they did not. In any
case her doctors didn't think that could account for her severe
depression and anxiety. The psychiatrist kept adding more drugs
to try to control her symptoms. Eventually she was able to return
to school on a cocktail of six or eight drugs: something to help
her concentrate, something to keep her awake, something to
help her sleep, something for depression, and something for

anxiety, along with oral contraceptives. Still, she felt nothing like her old self. "If it weren't for my family," she told me, "I would have died."

AN INCIDENTAL FINDING

In 1987, researchers organized a conference in Denver that was among the first of its kind—one that brought scientists studying fragile X syndrome together with affected families. Mothers of children with fragile X syndrome were interested in learning something about their children's rare condition. In turn, researchers had something to learn from mothers.

Because the mutated gene that caused fragile X syndrome was not identified until 1991, in 1987 mothers of children with fragile X disorders were considered "obligate carriers"—meaning that the laws governing X-linkage showed that they *must* be carriers, since that was the only way they could have children with fragile X syndrome. Obligate carriers were subdivided into those with or those without mental impairment—more specifically, intellectual disability. We now know that those *with* intellectual disability were mostly not premutation carriers, but women with the full mutation. Those without intellectual disability were more likely to be fragile X premutation carriers.

One session at the conference focused on fragile X syndrome and family planning. Mothers of kids with fragile X syndrome would be interested in options for having more children *without* fragile X, or so researchers thought. Genetic epidemiologist Stephanie Sherman recalls that at that Denver meeting, obligate carriers attended a discussion group on planning for future pregnancies.[4]

In this informal setting, one woman commented that the subject wasn't really relevant for her, as she had already been through menopause. Since she was under forty years old, in most settings this would be an isolated case of "premature menopause," which affects about 1 percent of women under forty. But to everyone's surprise, another young woman spoke up and told the group that she, too, had been through menopause. So did several more. Sherman and the others leading the workshop recognized the potential significance of this unexpected cohort of young women in menopause: a previously unrecognized effect of the mutated *FMR1* gene. "So we went off-topic!"

Genetic counselor Amy Cronister was at the workshop. She now studies cancer genetics at Integrated Genetics in Phoenix, Arizona, but in 1987 she was part of the team that had organized the conference. Cronister told me, "You have to remember, back in the '80s, before we were so overwhelmed with genetic information, what we really had to offer was important psychological and psychosocial support for fragile X families. . . . It was intimate and exhausting. We'd sit in the hallways, the families would absorb, and the clinicians would listen." At the time of the Denver conference in 1987, she added, "I said that's interesting, but heterozygotes [as carriers were then known] don't have symptoms." Faced with unexpected evidence to the contrary, Cronister set out to learn more about early menopause in heterozygotes. "For any genetic condition, if clinicians will really listen to their patients, it is amazing what can be discovered."[5]

Working with the Denver-based fragile X lab after the conference, Cronister surveyed obligate carriers, publishing her
findings in 1991.[6] She found that eight out of sixty-one, or 13 percent, of mentally unimpaired obligate carriers had had early
menopause (defined as cessation of menses before age forty).
None of the mentally impaired obligate carriers had had early
menopause.

Once the *FMR1* gene had been discovered in 1991, it was
possible to distinguish between women with the full mutation
and those who were premutation carriers.[7] It became clear that
premutation carriers, but not women with fragile X syndrome,
were at risk for premature menopause. As more was learned
about the condition, the name was changed: first to premature
ovarian failure, and finally to *fragile X–associated primary ovarian insufficiency,* or FXPOI, as it is now known. (It's pronounced
"FAX-POY.") Experts now recognize that approximately 20–
25 percent of carrier women will develop primary ovarian insufficiency. For patients with primary ovarian insufficiency (POI)
of unknown cause, approximately 2 percent with sporadic (non-
familial) and 14 percent with familial POI will turn out to be
FMR1 premutation carriers.[8]

Primary ovarian insufficiency is defined formally as cessation
of menses for four months in a woman under forty, with two
blood levels of follicle-stimulating hormone in the menopausal
range.[9] (Follicle-stimulating hormone interacts with the ovary
and causes an egg to be prepared for fertilization.) It affects
1 percent of US women under forty, 0.1 percent of women under
thirty, and .01 percent of women under age twenty. The average age at menopause for women in the United States is

fifty-one, but women with fragile X–associated primary ovarian insufficiency differ from the average menopausal woman in a number of ways.

In addition to the possibility of amenorrhea before age forty, which occurs in about a quarter of premutation carriers, women with the premutation experience menopause, on average, five to seven years earlier than women without a premutation. Some young women with a premutation may never establish normal periods but go on oral contraceptive pills as young teenagers to regulate heavy bleeding or irregularity (often further masking their lack of established menses). Even premutation women who menstruate regularly may experience decreased fertility, have higher follicle-stimulating hormone levels, and have fewer healthy ovarian follicles available to ripen should they opt for fertility treatment. Carriers are more likely to have ovarian cysts and to give birth to twins, a sign of ovarian dysfunction.[10]

Poorly functioning or nonfunctioning ovaries are unable to produce adequate estrogen. As a result of their chronic low-estrogen state, premutation women with primary ovarian insufficiency are susceptible to bone loss, falls, fractures, and cardiovascular disease and higher all-cause mortality,[11] and they may even be at higher risk of developing cognitive impairment as they age.[12]

Studies have found associations between POI and numerous other conditions in premutation carriers. One study compared carriers with POI to those without POI, along with unaffected controls. The study found that premutation carriers with POI had higher total rates of any immune-mediated disorders, defined in this study as autoimmune thyroid disease, fibromyalgia, irritable bowel syndrome, Raynaud's phenomenon, rheumatoid arthritis, Sjögren's syndrome, lupus, multiple sclerosis, and optic neuritis.[13] Another research group that reviewed the preexisting literature available on premutation carriers and health showed that premutation carriers with endocrine diseases—such as POI—were over six times more likely than carriers with no endocrine difficulties to report four or more serious medical problems. They reported more pain and used more analgesics. The authors concluded that carriers with endocrine dysfunction suffered from overall "ill health."[14]

After reviewing the literature, the authors of that study administered a questionnaire to a group of previously unstudied patients of their own. The group with endocrine problems was more likely to report neurologic symptoms like headache, tremor, and obsessive-compulsive disorder. Fibromyalgia occurred in carriers with endocrine problems, and not at all in those without endocrine problems.

SCREAMING TO THE OVARIES

Dr. Lawrence M. "Doc" Nelson is a retired public health officer of the National Institutes of Health who has devoted his career to the study and treatment of primary ovarian insufficiency. He is a widely recognized expert on POI. His 2009 invited article on the topic in the *New England Journal of Medicine* is considered authoritative.[15] His work at the National Institutes of Health and beyond stresses a holistic, integrated approach to the woman with ovarian insufficiency of any cause, recognizing that for some women it is a devastating diagnosis that changes their entire life's meaning.

Nelson reframes primary ovarian insufficiency as more than early menopause and possible infertility: it is a rare, serious, chronic disease with no cure. He characterizes a healthy menstrual cycle as a "vital sign" for young women's emotional and physical health. As such, POI requires an integrated, multispecialty approach to diagnosis and treatment, with an emphasis on adaptation to the diagnosis.

Nelson did a residency in obstetrics and gynecology at the University of Southern California. There he developed an interest in reproductive endocrinology. Back in the 1970s, there was no in-vitro fertilization, so options for treatment of infertility were limited. He set up an office in Lynchburg, Virginia, as a generalist, where he practiced for eight years. In the early 1980s he had a chance to evaluate a young woman with infertility and found she had a high level of follicle-stimulating hormone, or FSH, a level usually found in menopause. That same patient also had autoimmune thyroid disease. Nelson wondered if her ovaries could have been attacked by her own immune system. If so, suppressing her immune system safely might restore her fertility.

Convinced he was onto something, Nelson arranged for a research fellowship in London, where he learned research techniques under Robert Winston, a polymath and fertility expert in London who is now a baron, television personality, and member of the House of Lords. Nelson followed up with a fellowship studying autoimmune ovarian insufficiency at George

Washington University. When he finished his training, the National Institutes of Health was looking for a gynecologist to lead their research program. Nelson took the job and stayed for thirty years.

"No one is interested in a rare disease that doesn't kill you," Nelson told me.[16] I might add: and that doesn't affect men. (Most doctors, and even many gynecologists with whom I have spoken, are not aware of FXPOI, even though the diagnosis has been appreciated for over thirty years.) But the NIH was an ideal environment for research into rare diseases. They had the funds and were willing to look under every rock. There is an old saw still taught in medical school, "If you hear hoofbeats, look for horses, not zebras," meaning that common diagnoses are most commonly the right answer to a diagnostic question. "We were all curious research types looking for zebras," Nelson recalled. "We created a little pond, and all the big animals came and drank at our pond."

"Not that much has changed," he continued, in terms of the medical understanding and management of POI since Nelson wrote that journal article in 2009. He now devotes himself to helping patients find a new model of care. "We need to change the game."

For Nelson, the suicide of a patient with POI was a "wake-up call." Court documents related to her death contained diary entries that suggested that infertility was a significant factor in her suicide. It was at this point that Nelson began to change his approach to POI.

A bit over seventy at this writing, Nelson is tall, loose-limbed, and bearded. He still wears his NIH uniform (the National

Institutes of Health is a uniformed services organization, like the Navy), his hat and stripes and military bearing, when giving a lecture, but most of the time his mood is light, even goofy. His playfulness takes him wherever he needs to go on behalf of his patients, from Lakota shamanism to filmmaking. His creed is that medicine needs to be scientifically based, but also that physicians need to be engaged through their passions and emotions.[17]

Nelson's passions are diverse; for example, he is making a film that highlights George Washington's consequential decision to inoculate his troops against smallpox, which he argues just may have won the Revolutionary War. As far as POI is concerned, Nelson believes that the way research is currently conducted is not as beneficent as it should be, since women with POI are not generally considered important stakeholders in scientific research. Instead, they are subjects, and their data, including samples of their bodies and of their inner lives, is owned by researchers. He advocates a different model of care. This is what he means by "changing the game."

One woman described her experience in the NIH's 2008 inpatient study of POI for a medical journal: "While at the NIH, I met with at least ten medical professionals, including an endocrinologist, nutritionist, psychiatrist, occupational therapist, recreational therapist, spiritual counselor, and the Principal Investigator (LMN)—a reproductive endocrinologist by training. Not to mention the phlebotomists and sonographers! Each explored a different aspect of my wellbeing."[18]

Another "graduate" of the NIH's protocol, Daisy, went into more detail in an email to me:

Going to NIH was a true lifesaver for me. We had a room-
mate, and we were on different test schedules, so we could
tell each other what to expect from each test. Lots of blood-
work over the 3 days. I remember an ultrasound of the ovaries, bone density test, depression screening and talking with
a psychiatrist, talking with either a life coach/ occupational
therapist/ psychologist (I don't remember what the position
was called, but it was someone that really talked about our
aspirations and dreams for the future, work, and focus).

At the end of the 3 days, [Dr. Nelson] met with my
roomie and myself and our partners . . . and then myself
and partner alone. . . . During the group session, he went
over what all the tests were looking for, why each test was
done and how they relate to each other, and overall care
and wellbeing. He discussed what POI was, and related
conditions, and how the endocrine system works and how
different hormones play off each other (for example, POI is
identified from high FSH levels—well, I learned that the
FSH is the hormone that tells the ovaries to release the
egg; if the ovary isn't working correctly, FSH "shouts"
louder to try and be heard, and it's a vicious cycle—which
is why FSH levels can rise and rise, because it is literally
screaming to the ovaries to release the eggs. In the individual session, he went into the results of every test, and
the meaning of every result.[19]

Perhaps most important for a young woman like Daisy or Ariel
is for her healthcare team to recognize that receiving a diagnosis
of FXPOI, or any form of POI for that matter, can be an

emotional roller-coaster that for many women requires a reexamination of what gives their lives meaning.

Studies at NIH and elsewhere have found that loss of purpose in life is significantly associated with depression and anxiety, and a sense of purpose in life with resilience.[20] Women newly diagnosed with POI must undergo a "psychosocial transition" to a new sense of purpose—one not centered on childbearing—in order to get and stay well. To start, the low self-esteem so often experienced by women with diminished fertility needs to be addressed. In Nelson's view, health begins with destigmatization and avoidance of terms like "ovarian failure."

"Based on my interaction with teens and young women who get this diagnosis," Nelson wrote, "this is how I believe they hear these terms: 'You have premature MENOPAUSE! You have premature ovarian FAILURE! You have premature ovarian AGING!' These are stigmatizing and frightening terms to girls and young women."[21]

Women newly diagnosed with POI were surveyed and reported the following concerns in order of frequency: infertility, sexual life, taking hormone replacement therapy, fatigue, confidence, body image, poor memory, sexual partner, weight gain, low self-image, stress, overall health, joint pain, and headache. Their worries about all of these potential problems made the diagnosis a psychological minefield, and all wanted more support that was appropriate to their age.[22]

A high incidence of depression has been reported in women with POI, with a lifetime rate of major depressive disorder of 54 percent in POI as opposed to 20 percent in the National Co-morbidity Survey, a large community study of mental illness in the general population.[23] For many women, the onset of depression occurred after they had developed symptoms of POI, but before they were properly diagnosed, as in Ariel's case. Ariel was ill for three years and consulted numerous specialists before being diagnosed back in 2006. Even in 2019, a study based in Newark, New Jersey, reported that for urban women, many of color, the mean time from the onset of symptoms of POI to a proper diagnosis was six years![24]

Nelson advocates the model of "communities of practice" developed by social theorist Etienne Wenger during the late 1990s.[25] A community of practice—for example, a miscellaneous group of interested parties, both professionals and patients, who care about FXPOI or someone who has it—shares knowledge and has leaders who don't get bogged down in biases and fixed agendas. It pays attention to the physical, mental, emotional, and spiritual dimensions of health, by focusing on what it *means* to be a part of this community.

Writing about his own experience as a patient with prostate cancer, oncologist I.A. Roos described the online community of practice he joined, from which he learned "my *patientry*; in which I could negotiate meaning, and claim my new identity as a cancer patient."[26] Doc Nelson has started a closed Facebook group, My Family Cares about Primary Ovarian Insufficiency and Early Menopause, that addresses these same issues. Patients express themselves openly, respond to one another, and get gentle, nonjudgmental guidance from Doc about *how to help themselves*. By learning to help themselves, patients with POI claim new identities—as women with POI, who live with POI but are not defined by it. That is their "psychosocial transition."

As Daisy told me, "not having kids is a whole different set of challenges, but also opportunities, that not many people take the time to talk about. I refer to myself as childfree by circumstance—happy to be childfree, but honoring the struggle I went through to get to where I am now."

A HAPPY ENDING

Ariel's case was a "classic zebra." Luckily for Ariel, her mother's investment in all things fragile X had led to a personal friendship with Stephanie Sherman. After hearing about Ariel's misery, Stephanie felt she should talk over her history with Doc Nelson and other experts from the National Institutes of Health in a conference call, which Ariel was reluctant to do. She had reason to feel hopeless about doctors; none of them had done a thing for her, and she believed that one of the medications a psychiatrist had prescribed had made her feel suicidal. She no longer trusted physicians. "I just started hating doctors, I have distrust of them still." But to please her mother, she agreed to speak to a team of researchers and clinicians from the National Institutes of Health. Ariel was disgusted when one asked her if she had tried meditation. "I called my mom, and told her I didn't like that conversation. But that man was Dr. Nelson."[27]

With his knowledge of primary ovarian insufficiency in general, and fragile X–associated primary ovarian insufficiency in particular, Nelson could have made Ariel's diagnosis over the phone. Instead, he says, "We invited her to come to the pond."

She had no interest in doing so, but Belle bribed her with the promise of a "girls' weekend," just the two of them. When the hospital bracelet was placed around Ariel's wrist, she felt betrayed and panicky, but the evaluation was brief. An FSH level was drawn, and Ariel met with a psychiatrist, who surmised that her depression and anxiety were related to hormonal disarray and the preceding three years with no diagnosis and a constant influx of misinformation. The blood level confirmed ovarian insufficiency. By 2006, Ariel, now twenty, had undergone a three-year diagnostic odyssey despite having a brother with fragile X syndrome and a known diagnosis of the premutation. Her ordeal changed her life, her family's lives, and her doctor's life, and it had an impact on the future of rare disease diagnosis and management.

Ariel was put on physiologic hormone replacement (which is different from either the contraceptive pill or the type of replacement used by older women with natural menopause), and gradually, over several weeks, she felt better and better. On estrogen patches and progesterone pills in the right sequence, she was raring to return to college, "in a state of like, 'FREEDOM!'"

Ariel is both well-adjusted and lucky. Lucky to have a loving, determined mother with means and social connections. Lucky to be thrilled, not devastated, by a diagnosis of ovarian insufficiency, for which treatment allowed her to return to the productive and cheerful person she had always been. At twenty, Ariel wasn't interested in having children; she wanted to have fun. I also think she's lucky in character: her years of depression and anxiety are for her a big blur with a good explanation, not a trauma she returns to and mourns. When I asked her in an email how she put the unhappiness behind her, she wrote: "It saddens me that I had to have three very, very, very shitty years, but I am glad I finally got a diagnosis. I was getting scared that I would have to live the rest of my life like that."[28]

Ariel has been exceptionally lucky, too, in that like 5–10 percent of women diagnosed with ovarian insufficiency and properly treated with hormones, she has been able to conceive and bear children. She chose to terminate her first pregnancy when she learned that the fetus she was carrying had fragile X syndrome. Though she feared it might be the only time she ever got pregnant, Ariel had no reservations about terminating the pregnancy. "I love my brother," she told me, "but that's not the life I want to live."

It took four more years of trying before she was pregnant again. "My husband said he had 'super-sperm,' getting an infertile woman pregnant." Sperm can live in the fallopian tubes for two to three days, and women struggling to conceive are often advised to have sex three times a week to keep themselves loaded with viable sperm in case an egg is released from an ovary. "It put pressure on our relationship, for sure," Ariel said, but finally she was pregnant, and she and her husband sweated out what they came to call the "maybe baby" trimester. Maybe they would have a baby. Or maybe they would choose to abort another fragile X fetus. They got lucky, again, and had their first daughter, and a few years later, another girl. When we spoke, Ariel was pregnant again, in the earliest weeks, and an ultrasound had shown an empty sac. "I'm 99 percent sure

I'm miscarrying," she told me, "but I still feel kinda pumped. My ovary did something!"

RISKS

The American College of Obstetrics and Gynecology (ACOG) notes that POI is a disease state and is not equivalent to a hastening of natural menopause. The recommended regimen of hormone replacement differs from that for women with natural menopause.

POI does require treatment with hormone replacement therapy to reduce the risk of osteoporosis, cardiovascular disease, and urogenital atrophy and to improve quality of life. ACOG recommends that women with POI be treated with hormone replacement therapy until they are fifty-one years old, the average age at menopause.[29] Approximately 5–10 percent of women with POI can conceive naturally, since up to 50 percent of women with POI ovulate intermittently. Oral contraceptives can actually improve fertility in POI, since they tend to lower FSH levels.

The cause for most cases of POI is never determined. The most common *genetic* cause, however, is the *FMR1* premutation, known to be responsible for about 6 percent of cases of POI. FXPOI is a special type of POI in a number of ways.

Most significant for women with FXPOI is the possibility of having a child with fragile X syndrome. As Ariel did, a small but significant percentage of women with FXPOI can get pregnant, either spontaneously or with assisted reproductive technologies. Most women who develop FXPOI have enough CGG repeats that their likelihood of having a fragile X child approaches 100 percent if the child inherits the affected X chromosome. Without a known diagnosis of FXPOI, medical treatments of infertility can lead to the birth of a baby with fragile X syndrome. A National Institutes of Health case report documents the history of a young woman whose POI of unknown cause remitted with hormone replacement therapy. She conceived a child with assisted reproductive techniques, who was later discovered to have fragile X syndrome.[30] The woman had not been previously diagnosed with FXPOI, but testing after her daughter was born did reveal her to be a premutation carrier.

It seems likely that FXPOI has a similar mechanism to other premutation-related diseases that will be discussed in later chapters: toxic RNA related to CGG repeat length.[31] The fact that the majority of carrier women do *not* develop FXPOI suggests that it is a "polygenic" disorder, one that requires the presence of multiple different mutations.[32]

For some premutation conditions, the more CGG repeats a man or woman has, the more likely he or she is to develop the condition. But surprisingly, in FXPOI, the association is curvilinear, with a peak in the "mid-range" area and troughs on either side. In other words, women with 80–100 CGG repeats are at highest risk and at risk for the earliest onset of FXPOI. Thirty-two percent of women with 80–100 repeats will develop FXPOI,[33] but women with greater than 100 or fewer than 80 CGG repeats are less likely to develop it, and if they do, will develop it later in life.[34] Other high-risk groups include women with a family history of early ovarian insufficiency (age at meno-pause tends to be a familial trait) and women who smoke (this is true for non-fragile-X associated POI as well).

Medical management of FXPOI is essential, regardless of the woman's childbearing plans. The essence of treatment of FXPOI, as with idiopathic POI, is hormone replacement. And that, Nelson explains, should not just be oral contraceptives. These expose the woman to higher than normal levels of hor-mones. For Nelson, the ideal regimen was developed at NIH as a result of their intensive study of women with POI.[35] Women should begin hormone replacement as soon as they receive a diagnosis of POI and continue beyond their childbearing years until the average age of menopause.

Ariel is a case in point: as a twenty-year-old with POI, she had the bone density of an eighty-year-old woman. A few years later, at follow-up, her bone density had returned to normal thanks to hormone replacement.

MAYBE BABY

Complicating the situation for women with FXPOI in partic-ular, in a survey by reproductive endocrinologist Heather Hipp and her colleagues of seventy-nine women with FXPOI at her Emory University–based clinic, the mean age of onset of FXPOI was thirty-three years of age, with over half of these women already coping with having at least one child with frag-ile X syndrome. They benefited, perhaps due to their known premutation carrier status, with a time to diagnosis of only about one year. Nonetheless, over half of them had had inadequate to no hormone replacement and had osteoporosis or low bone mineral density. Many were deeply conflicted between the joy their fragile X child had brought them and their desire to have another child without the syndrome.[36]

I had a chance to visit Hipp in her office at Emory University Hospital, which overlooks the imposing Atlanta skyline. She told me how hard it was to give women with FXPOI such a bum diagnosis. Because the diagnosis requires laboratory testing, it can't be made at the first visit. There is just no good way to do it. She calls some women on the phone, which catches many at work or in the car and can seem insensitive, and she emails others who don't want to be called during a busy and unpredictable day, though some women find that totally heartless. "Ideally you'd bring them back to the office for some 'news'—but most women can't wait that long."

She would like to start these conversations by emphasizing the importance of hormone replacement therapy, but generally patients with FXPOI are urgently preoccupied with getting pregnant, not taking hormones. In addition, she has noticed something about women with FXPOI in particular: when I asked what it was like to be with women with FXPOI versus women with autoimmune or idiopathic POI, she hesitated. "It's not tangible . . . more women are tangential, they seem to have higher levels of affective disorders, they spend a lot of time talking."[37] You might think that could apply to anyone with POI, but Hipp says that others on her team have noticed and will often identify carriers with FXPOI by the way they speak. Another researcher at the Emory Clinic told me that if questions were not structured, women with FXPOI would go off-topic in a way she had never noticed with mothers of kids with Down syndrome, who seem more able to focus. "They're very all-over-the-place," she told me.[38]

It may be that learning differences common to premutation women make the diagnosis even more difficult to absorb and to respond to in an organized way. Nonetheless, Hipp's article noted, many women with FXPOI practiced self-advocacy: "During the interviews, several women who knew their carrier status reported printing out information from fragile X websites and taking it to their gynecologist after their initial concerns were discounted."[39]

For women with FXPOI who want to have children, there are a handful of options.[40] Ariel and her husband were fortunate to conceive naturally, and to follow up with prenatal testing and in the case of her first pregnancy, termination of a fragile X pregnancy. She now has two unaffected daughters. For some women, natural conception is a possibility, but termination is not acceptable to them; these women may forego prenatal testing or choose to do it without opting for termination.

Options for prenatal testing are invasive; the *FMR1* mutation can't be detected in the fetus by sampling the mother's blood or cheek swab. Instead, the mother can have chorionic villus sampling, or CVS, at 10.5 to 11.5 weeks gestation. A small sample of the placenta is taken through the mother's cervix. Results are available in three days.

Another method is amniocentesis, which can be performed from fifteen to eighteen weeks of gestation. A few tablespoons of amniotic fluid are removed from the uterus and require three weeks to grow in a culture medium. This test can be used to give more genetic information, but it has the obvious disadvantage of occurring much later in pregnancy.

Assisted reproductive technologies include using a donor egg. The donor's eggs are harvested after hormonal priming and fertilized, typically with the affected mother's partner's sperm. After five days the tiny embryo is placed in the mother's uterus.

The most complicated and costly procedure is in vitro fertilization with preimplantation genetic diagnosis. Here a fertility center harvests eggs from the affected mother. This can be a challenge, or in fact impossible, given the mother's limited ovarian function, but in some cases it is successful. The egg is fertilized, and the resulting embryos are frozen at the 6–8 cell stage. The embryos are then sent to one of the few sites in the world that is able to do *FMR1* testing by biopsy. A cell or two can be removed at this early stage and tested for *FMR1* mutations. Only an embryo negative for *FMR1* mutations will then be returned to the mother for implantation and gestation. This option, if successful, produces a child biologically related to both parents without an *FMR1* mutation and no need for termination; however, it is beyond the financial means of many would-be parents.

Some younger women who know their fragile X premutation status may choose to freeze their eggs or an embryo at a young age, before they are ready to have children, with the idea that they might lose their fertility by the time they can commit to parenthood. Nelson highly recommends this method, since ovarian function can continue to deteriorate over time.[41]

Finally, a couple can choose adoption or not to have children at all.

CHANGING THE GAME

If Ariel were to search for a silver lining hidden inside those three "very, very, very shitty years," she could take comfort in knowing that her journey from hopeless shut-in to brave young mother was brought to bear on at least a couple of major innovations in health care delivery.

Ariel's eldest brother, Franklin, nine years older than she, was not genotypically affected by fragile X mutations, but thanks to James, he had lived with fragile X most of his life. Already grown up and living away from home when Ariel was in a wretched state of depression and anxiety, he remained close to his family and was shocked by Ariel's increasing debilitation.

In hindsight, he now says, it was obvious that she had FXPOI, but at the time, "her diagnoses were just descriptions of her symptoms."[42] Franklin described himself to me as "a serial entrepreneur"—a venture capitalist always on the lookout for opportunities to succeed in tech. Ariel's diagnostic journey provided inspiration. She had been diagnosed with a rare disease when she brought herself to the National Institutes of Health to be evaluated by ten professionals who put their diverse perspectives and experiences together to solve a problem. Rather than bring the patient to the experts, Franklin wondered, why couldn't the internet be used to bring unlimited expertise to the patient?

Franklin had read James Surowiecki's book *The Wisdom of Crowds*, an influential 2004 book about crowdsourcing and how it shapes economies and societies.[43] Surowiecki argued that crowds could be "smarter" than experts so long as the individuals within the crowd were diverse, thought independently of one another, and were decentralized, without an authoritarian structure. In the special case of science, Surowiecki pointed out, scientists were in competition with one another to make discoveries, but the scientific process required cooperation through publication. "Scientists were paid by other people's attention," he writes.[44] In other words, if scientists kept their work secret and did not allow others to see their methods and conclusions, they would never receive credit for the work they had done.

"This tradition of open publication and communication of insights was, of course, central to the success of Western science," Surowiecki adds. "It's open science that made the self-interested behavior of scientists collectively beneficial. Scientists were willing to publish their insights because that was the route to public recognition and influence." In other words, Western science has evolved as a form of crowdsourcing, with each lab working independently, using its own quirks and strengths, and communicating with others across the world.

Surowiecki gave the medical example of SARS, the *severe acute respiratory syndrome*, which emerged in Asia in 2003. The World Health Organization suspected a viral cause and asked eleven labs from all over the world to cooperate in identifying it. The labs shared their findings with each other, but each worked independently. They identified the virus within a few weeks. Surowiecki noted, "The intriguing thing about the success of the laboratories' collaboration is that no one, strictly speaking, was in charge of it."[45] The labs racing to find the cause of SARS were diverse, independent, and decentralized—an ideal "crowd" that was smarter than any single expert.

Franklin believed that Ariel could have benefited from crowd wisdom. She had spent three years consulting experts. Like Ariel, Franklin had become cynical. "Patients have blind trust in doctors. They think the medical system is there to help them. That's just not the case."[46]

What if diverse individuals, working independently, with no one in charge, had been able to bring their talents to bear on her diagnostic dilemma? This was the inspiration for Crowd-Med, an online game that doctors, medical students, and other rare-disease nerds play for money while patients gamble that the crowd can do what none of their doctors have been able to do: diagnose their disease. Patients pay about $500 to present their cases, and they complete and upload what Franklin called "an intake form on steroids"—personal and family histories, lab and other test results, notes from prior consultations, and so on. Then the case is "exposed" to the crowd.

Gamers can brainstorm together, share opinions, and propose diagnoses, and can chat with patients. All communications are available to all. Gamers are rated with a "reputation score" based on their qualifications and past performances, which allows their diagnoses to rise to the top of the list, only to be replaced by other, more likely diagnoses that the crowd can select should they be suggested. Eventually the case is closed, and the patient has thirty days to choose the best answer and to let CrowdMed know if the diagnosis was medically confirmed. The patient decides how to divide a cash reward to the most helpful players.

For a trial run, in 2013, Franklin used Ariel's medical records. Seven years had passed since her diagnosis, but little had changed in terms of the average doctor's awareness of the condition. Twenty to thirty diagnoses were proposed within three weeks. The most compelling was FXPOI.

Chapter Five

THE MOVEMENT DISORDER THAT
STARTED A MOVEMENT

FRAGILE X–ASSOCIATED TREMOR/ATAXIA
SYNDROME (FXTAS)

MEN IN their fifties and sixties don't come to a pediatrician's office complaining of tremor, gait disturbance, and personality changes. It was their daughters, visiting the office with their kids, who piqued Randi Hagerman's interest in grandfathers.

Randi's devotion to children with fragile X syndrome, and their mothers, has meant the world to their families (see chapter 1). But in academic medicine, she is more likely to be remembered for her identification of FXTAS (pronounced FAX-TASS), a disease of mostly older men.

A DISTRACTING DRAIN

The Kellers live in a spacious, snug compound in southern Oregon: two houses surrounded by trees, an enormous garage, and lots of room for safe play.[1] Zach Keller, fifteen, was diagnosed with fragile X syndrome as a baby, and although he is severely affected by autism, he is the adored flag-bearer of his high school band, doted upon by neighborhood girls. His parents stress that he has *earned* his popularity through positive behaviors, hard work in therapy and at school, and innate goodness.

Liv and Jonathan downplay their own role in his achievements, but it is clear that without their insistence on good behavior and friendliness, Zach would not be a beloved local celebrity. Liv's devotion to Zach's social skills is a vocation, exhausting at times, but compelling and worthwhile. On the other hand, there is her father, Dave, whose struggles with acceptable behavior are a distracting drain. Dave lives with Liv's mother in the compound's smaller home.

Dave is seventy, but he looks like an aged baby—a wise old dumpy gnome in a wheelchair. He can't walk any more, thanks to a listing gait, frequent falls, and, perhaps most of all, lack of motivation to get around. He has the fragile X–associated tremor/ataxia syndrome—FXTAS—a degenerative neurologic disorder that may afflict up to 75 percent of male carriers of fragile X syndrome.[2]

The tremor associated with FXTAS is an intention tremor, which is most obvious when an affected individual is doing something purposeful with his hands, like picking up a teacup or putting a key into a lock. Ataxia refers to a drunken, uncoordinated swaying motion that affects walking and other movements. But FXTAS may be most notable for the personality changes it causes as the disease becomes apparent.

About a year before Zach was born, there was a strange and memorable incident. Dave's wife, Annie, had stocked the pantry with a big load of toilet paper from Costco. When she went to get some for the bathroom, it was gone. When she inquired about it, Dave was defiant and hostile. "That's my toilet paper," he told her. "If you want some, go buy your own."[3] Perplexed, Annie searched the house and found the paper hidden behind his shirts.

Dave had been a sociable project manager, a man who could visualize solutions, make plans, prioritize, and get things done—a good executive. In FXTAS, an impairment of these "executive functions" is often the first thing people notice. Dave seemed to lose interest in just about everything, content to stay in his room all day watching game shows and insulting his wife. If he went out, he might come back from a restaurant bathroom with a toilet seat cover wrapped around his neck, like a scarf. Though he explained that it was a joke, no one else thought it was funny. By the time Zach was diagnosed with fragile X syndrome a couple of years later, Dave was depressed and increasingly socially isolated, complaining of pain in his back and legs.

As Zach grew up, Dave continued to deteriorate. "In comparison to the dad who raised me, he's nowhere near the same guy," said Liv. He can't really follow a train of thought, and little events that require adaptation, like the change from daylight time to standard, completely confuse him. Still, Liv thinks that some of his decline is volitional. "He likes to pee in a coffee can, but he can walk into Waffle House and order food when he feels like it." She demands that he remember his dignity, just as she insists that Zach remember his manners, but she has made a lot more headway with Zach.

When Dave was finally diagnosed with FXTAS—not by a neurologist, but by Zach's pediatrician—it explained a lot.

RESONATING

I first interviewed Randi Hagerman in 2015, and my visit to the Kellers was part of a longer visit to the western states in November 2016, which culminated in several days at MIND Institute.

Her office at the MIND Institute, at the university's medical center in Sacramento, is cluttered, and files are hard to find, but Randi has a photographic memory for the DNA variations (genotypes) and physical features (phenotypes) of the innumerable children she has seen over the past forty years. I was able to page through some of those files. Randi's notes documented thoughtful and loving observations of fragile X kids. One in particular stayed with me. Describing a little boy with fragile X syndrome, she wrote, "When he is angry, he raises his fist in the Black Power salute."

That sentence told me a lot about Randi. She grew up in the Bay Area during the 1960s. She had a sense of humor. But more important for a doctor, she had a lively imagination that she could call upon to see patients differently. She used her own life experience to organize her assessment. She noticed the child's behavior and connected it to a feeling. She admired her patient, and she trusted her own impressions.

The rugged, bony daughter of a Norwegian sea captain, Randi grew up in Berkeley, chasing her brothers around while their mother worked. Seventy at this writing, Randi still has enough energy to control a roomful of hyperactive fragile X boys while soothing their mothers and training aspiring pediatricians at the same time. She travels incessantly—to Iran, India, Israel, Jordan, Saudi Arabia, Argentina, and the Philippines in a single year—while conducting research in California. She is never idle, dyeing her own clothes and making prints during her downtime. On a rare vacation, she climbed Mount Kilimanjaro.[4]

But what had made me want to meet Randi was to learn how this woman scientist had discovered a significant, devastating, previously unrecognized neurologic disease with a unique mechanism of action through conversation with mothers. It was resonating with other women that led to the discovery of FXTAS. And it was having the tools—self-confidence and drive—to "sell" the diagnosis to other physicians that led to its acceptance in mainstream medicine.

THE HAGERMANS ON TOUR

Randi Hagerman is the world's foremost expert in fragile X disorders. Her husband, Paul Hagerman, is an honored academic scientist who studies the molecular biology of fragile X disorders at the Davis research campus (figure 5.1). At grand rounds all over the world, Randi gets a laugh by calling Paul "Daddy," while he rolls his eyes, relishing—at least in public—the role of beleaguered sidekick.

A little showmanship is required to snare busy physicians and bring them into the field, from which Randi has sworn she will

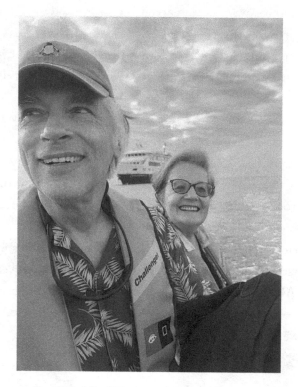

FIGURE 5.1 Randi and Paul Hagerman. Photographer unknown, 2021. Photo courtesy of Randi Hagerman.

never retire until someone finds a cure for fragile X. It's also required to maintain the attention of intellectually disabled children and adults. In the world of fragile X kids and their parents, she has movie-star charisma.

Having seen her in action, I can say this about Randi Hagerman: there is something unusually powerful about the way she connects with people. And it's not just patients. She has vastly increased awareness of fragile X disorders in pediatricians, neurologists, obstetricians, and bench researchers through charisma and persuasion. When Randi and Paul Hagerman gave a talk to first-year medical students at the University of California, Davis, I sat in.[5]

Randi went first and took up most of the hour, illustrating her talk with pictures of families and video clips of kids flying into a rage when she approached, demonstrating "tactile defensiveness"—the tendency of fragile X children to resist being touched. She explained that fragile X boys nearly all have marked enlargement of their testes when they reach puberty—and sometimes, still in infancy—and showed some startling photographs of boys with huge balls, accompanied by a good yarn about a nonclinical social worker recoiling in amazement from what he saw when asked to help out with a child's diaper. The students laughed, in part at the social worker's expense, but that was okay because he wasn't there. Of course, they were also laughing because little boys' genitals made them nervous. Randi's joke helped defuse the tension, but later she told me it had another purpose.

"They won't forget what they saw," she explained. "I've got to capture people's interest or I'll never be able to retire." She knows that fragile X syndrome is a rare disease, an "orphan" disease that still needs to prove its value to researchers, drug companies, and medical students, most of whom will never see a child with fragile X syndrome. Medical students have many competing priorities, but this lecture was an opportunity to turn them on to the fragile X field. If her life's work is to continue, she needs to inspire more doctors and researchers.

When Randi and Paul lecture together, they have another bit of shtick—Paul groans at Randi's intrusion into his lecture time and rolls his eyes, playing the role of henpecked Dr. Hagerman, once again pushed around by his wife, Dr. Hagerman. The students are absolutely charmed. They ask questions enthusiastically. After the lecture, many more surround Paul. He's the affable, accessible first mate to the ship's captain, and as such he draws a crowd, even though his material is more difficult and abstract. A distinguished molecular biologist whose work unpacks the process by which fragile X mutations wreak havoc on a microscopic level, Paul's slides were dense, but he's a clear speaker, and, I think even more important, offers surprised students an opportunity to reenter the world of hard science and get comfortable there. Randi and Paul together are so much more effective than either would be alone. Randi provides a lot of food for thought in an entertaining package, and Paul explicates and soothes. When the lectures are over, the students are excited about fragile X syndrome. They won't forget what they saw today, and they won't forget what they learned, either.

After the lecture, I followed Randi from the medical center to their home in my car. She took forever to finish up at her office, sharing stories with me. She loves to tell the story of how she met Paul—she pegged him as the smartest, best-looking man in their class at Stanford Medical School, and she went for it. "I had to steal him from all these East Coast women who wanted him," she laughed. They have two grown daughters now, and grandchildren from each. Off-campus, at least with a visitor present, they continue to enact the dynamic I saw at the medical center: Randi leads with a lot of passion, and Paul contributes something thoughtful, lucid, and memorable.

Paul called, asking her to get a move on. When we finally arrived at their home, Paul complained about her abuse of his time, as he had during the lecture; now, though, I had the feeling he was actually annoyed. But he had used the extra time to invent a new dish, fish in a sauce thickened with a secret ingredient, which Randi and I could not guess. It was crushed Fritos.

Randi and Paul are so *likeable*. I'm convinced that this has had a huge impact on the fragile X field, and it certainly has had an impact on the lives of patients and advocates who know them personally. Seeing patients with Randi, I was struck by her attentiveness to each member of the family and by her capacity to meet them where they are. She warmed up Todd, a wriggling fragile X four-year-old, by chatting with his parents and praising his speech ("Mama, sit!") before getting into his space. She stayed close just long enough to hear his heartbeat and look into his eyes, then got out of the way before he could whack her. His father, an entrepreneur, runs a business marketing medical marijuana, and they discussed the use of cannabinoids for fragile X-related anxiety. The boy's grandmother wasn't sure marijuana is good for kids, and Randi concurred. Todd's mother asked about antioxidants for her own stress management, and she and Randi discussed green tea and blueberries. Todd's babysitter was there, too; as his mother said warmly, "She is my wife." Randi gets that.

Logistic and financial pressures on doctors often lead them to spend limited time with families, entering data into electronic medical records. "I never do that!" Randi practically shouted. Good doctors don't, but good medical researchers don't either. FXTAS was discovered by clinicians who observed, heard, and cared about their patients, and by parents whose observations were taken seriously.

One instance: Liv and Jonathan Keller tried to learn everything they could about fragile X syndrome after Zach was diagnosed as a baby. He was frequently ill with high fevers. Jonathan went to a talk Randi gave at the National Fragile X Foundation in California. Afterward he approached her and said, "My son is very sick, and he needs you."

She was in the middle of a meeting, but Randi didn't hesitate. "Where is he?" She was ready to examine him on the spot.

That kind of devotion to patients—even to a baby she hadn't met yet—is what makes Randi a heroine to so many families. At some point, in response to Randi's evident curiosity and interest in the entire family, Liv mentioned her father's tremor, difficulty walking, and surprising transformation from successful project manager to irritable hoarder.

"PEOPLE THINK I GO OFF THE DEEP END"

The MIND Institute is now located at the University of California, Davis, but many of the clinicians and scientists who work there got their start at Denver Children's Hospital during the 1980s. At Denver Children's, Randi Hagerman came to mentor and through grants financially support a team of clinicians and scientists devoted to fragile X treatment and research

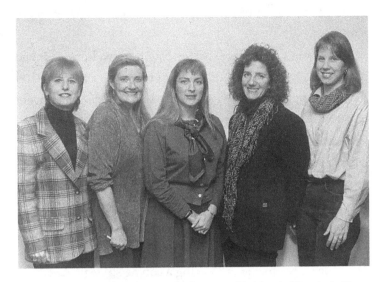

FIGURE 5.2 The clinical team at Denver Children's Hospital. From left to right: Louise Gane, Randi Hagerman, Rebecca O'Connor, Sarah Scharfenaker, and Tracy Stackhouse. Photographer unknown, mid-1990s.
Collection of Louise Gane.

(figure 5.2). Paul Hagerman conducted laboratory-based work, and occupational therapists, psychologists, and clinical researchers worked with kids. A genetic counselor, Louise Gane, joined the group in the early 1990s, and for families, she became as important a figure as Randi Hagerman was. Her emphasis was on not on "genetic" but on "counselor."

Where Randi was vigorous and optimistic, Louise was gentle and supportive. She has a soft, unplaceable accent that turns out to be that of a New Zealander who has lived in the United States for much of her adult life. She had—still has—a way of getting to the heart of the matter that makes you want to cry with her.

Louise was a qualified expert in fragile X syndrome, but one of her tasks at Denver Children's was to answer the phone and schedule appointments. This was partly because they were underfunded, and her secretarial services were part of the package, but it served another purpose: when a parent first reached out to Denver Children's with a new diagnosis of fragile X, the intervention could begin on the phone. "Often I was the first person they'd ever spoken to about fragile X. I'd make suggestions of how to talk to the teacher and how to talk to their local doctors about treatment. I'd normalize the diagnosis. They'd leave the phone call having a coping strategy. And consciously or unconsciously, I was recruiting for studies."[6]

During the last few years of the twentieth century, Louise noticed something. Mothers—the ones who were on the phone with her, trying to wrap their heads around the diagnosis of fragile X syndrome in their children—had questions about their fathers. Their fathers had changed, becoming irritable, irrational, and impulsive. Their wives and children watched helplessly as their behavior grew coarse and their movements clumsy. Could this be related to the fragile X gene?

Louise often interceded with the ever overextended Randi on behalf of patients. "I'd say, I don't think [it's related], but I will talk to Randi about it and tell you what she thinks." Randi always said no.

One day in the winter of 1999, yet another woman reached out to Louise for emotional support. Louise recalled, "She got to talking about her father, he was married, a leader in his community. All of a sudden he left his wife, married this young thing . . . he was impulsive, erratic with money. I remember talking to her and going to Randi with that question." Could this behavior—which, honestly, isn't unheard of in a middle-aged man—be caused by carrying an "asymptomatic" fragile X premutation?

That call was on top of five or six in quick succession. As Louise remembered it, Randi shrugged it off for a moment, as she always did, but then she stopped what she was doing and gave the question some thought. Finally she said, "Maybe this is something we should look into." Louise told me, "I literally said 'duh.'"[7]

Throughout the early 1990s Randi and Louise had noticed the recurrence of psychiatric complaints in mothers. It goes without saying that mothers of children with special needs face a hard road, often alone. They may spend more time with their children's doctors, therapists, and teachers than they do with any other adults, including their partners. At the MIND Institute, the long batteries of tests and extensive family history-taking brought mothers together with psychologists and genetic counselors over repeated visits. They began to notice a pattern: many of these mothers were depressed and anxious, which was no surprise, but they were also plagued by learning disabilities, migraines, sleep disorders, autoimmune conditions, some cancers, and early menopause. These carrier symptoms had never been given much attention by the research community.

"I could diagnose anxiety and depression by phone," Louise told me. She didn't mean by reviewing symptoms during the phone call, but by listening to the voices of the mothers. As I interviewed carrier mothers, I could see what she meant. There was a certain style, a frozen quality, which I heard over and over, as though a thin layer of ice kept an ocean of distress in check and the effort to keep it from shattering made the free expression of feelings impossible.

Randi and Louise knew that all mothers of fragile X kids are carriers. They hypothesized that beyond the stresses of raising children with fragile X syndrome, there was something about the carrier state itself that predisposed mothers to emotional disturbance.

"Moms would tell me about their emotional problems all the time," Randi told me, "and a lot of these problems predated their having kids with fragile X syndrome." Mothers commonly reported anxiety and difficulty maintaining eye contact. "People think I go off the deep end," Randi added, "but they don't take a holistic approach to medicine."[8]

Randi and Louise came to be certain that carriers were in fact different from noncarriers. But it was hard to get people outside the clinic to take their research seriously. Psychiatric problems were hard to define, subjective, vague—in neurological parlance, "soft." (See the next chapter.)

Very few scientists—actually, virtually none outside of the Hagermans and their crew—believed in carrier symptoms throughout the 1990s. Randi was told that psychiatric symptoms were impossible to attribute to the carrier state, and that what they had found was an artifact, a misleading effect of the act of examining a problem. Having it both ways, one reviewer for a medical journal told her, "This can't be right; if it were, somebody would have thought of it earlier."[9]

There was another, bigger obstacle to medically legitimizing carrier symptoms. The very definition of "carrier" is that while a carrier may be genetically anomalous, she is phenotypically normal, that is, normal as far as anyone can tell by looking. There should be no way to distinguish carriers, clinically, from noncarriers. Because by definition, fragile X carriers had no symptoms, researchers ignored data that contradicted this basic tenet of medical genetics.[10] In statistics, this error is known as *confirmation bias*. We see only what confirms what we already believe.

But mothers like Liv Keller hadn't read the same genetics textbooks. And she could see that something was very wrong with her father.

FXTAS

The first patient formally diagnosed with FXTAS at the MIND Institute was a retired firefighter named Clay who lived in Louisville, Kentucky. Clay's daughter, Jennifer, had a son with fragile X syndrome, which had been identified by Randi some years before.[11]

In his late fifties, Clay began to have tremor, listing to the side, and experienced falls. A gentle guy, he was far from irascible, but he had been forced to retire early because he couldn't work as a firefighter with such marked disabilities. He was diagnosed with Parkinson's disease. Nonetheless, he was optimistic about retirement, planning to build his own house outside Boulder, Colorado, where he loved the mountains. "He retired and he never got to do any of the things he wanted—bought all these tools for woodworking that he could not use," his daughter told me. He became more and more unsteady and began spending much of the day in a recliner in the living room. It was an effort to stand. He needed to be fed and became incontinent. Friends stopped visiting because it was too depressing. He became disoriented and had hallucinations.

When Jennifer told Randi her father's story, it fell on fertile soil. Randi and Louise had just had the conversation that ended when Louise said "Duh." Jennifer brought Clay to Randi's clinic, then in Denver. After talking to so many women about their fathers, Randi and Louise finally had a symptomatic grandfather in their clinic, a gentleman who was willing to undergo extensive testing. He even agreed to donate his brain upon his death. Soon, four more grandfathers had also agreed to be evaluated.

In June 2000, at the annual National Fragile X Foundation conference, Randi believed the time was right to discuss the five cases at a scientific meeting. The National Fragile X Foundation meetings are open to scientists, of course, and to families as well. For families adapting to life with rare diseases, meetings like these are a lifeline. Not only do they get to hear from experts, but they also meet other families who suffer from the same condition. A family with a fragile X child might otherwise never know another such family, and even their pediatrician might never have seen another child with fragile X syndrome.

But as with FXPOI, it turns out that in the case of FXTAS, the meetings were highly important to researchers as well.

"I thought this was rare," Randi recalled. "I asked the audience if they had ever seen anything like this in their own families. About a third to a half of the room raised their hands." Flora Tassone, a researcher in Paul's lab who was also at the meeting, remembers a woman standing up and saying, "You have described my father."[12] Stunned by this unexpected response, Randi and colleagues wrote up their five cases and submitted their article to the journal *Neurology*, where it was published in 2001.[13] Subsequently, for a 2004 case series, a fellow in the Hagerman lab, Sébastien Jacquemont, and Louise Gane visited every fragile X child's grandfather whom they could identify in the state of California. They presented twenty-six patients with the syndrome and formalized the criteria for FXTAS, including the presence of tremor, ataxia, cognitive and emotional changes, and specific MRI findings.

The combination of tremor, ataxia, and impaired judgment puts affected patients at risk of falling, as does the weakness and nerve damage often associated with FXTAS. Patients with FXTAS have lesions in both their brains and peripheral nerves, a combination that can make coordinating and executing everyday movements a huge challenge. The nerve damage is also associated with blood pressure abnormalities, erectile dysfunction, loss of bowel and bladder control, and chronic pain.

At the same time that diagnostic criteria were being worked out, researchers were trying to discover a mechanism of action for FXTAS: *why* it occurred, and in particular, why it might be associated with the premutation. The earliest hypothesis was that premutation-associated FMRP deficits—too little of the fragile X mental retardation protein—were likely to be causative, but Flora Tassone's research showed otherwise.

In 2000, Tassone, working with Paul Hagerman in his lab in Denver, had discovered excess *FMR1* messenger RNA (mRNA, one of many subtypes of RNA) in the blood of premutation carriers.[14] It was conceivable that too much mRNA lay behind the development of FXTAS symptoms. Carriers can have ten times as much *FMR1*-associated messenger RNA as noncarriers.

By definition, it will be recalled, while most people have around 30 CGG repeats in their *FMR1* genes, premutation carriers have anywhere between 55 and 199 CGG repeats. In both the premutation carrier and the full mutation fragile X individual, the coding part of the gene that makes FMRP is not altered. But there is a problem in the *regulation* of the gene; it *overworks* in the premutation carrier, transcribing too many copies of messenger RNA. This overwork allows premutation carriers to produce an adequate supply of FMRP, so premutation carriers don't have fragile X syndrome. Many of the problems faced by premutation carriers aren't caused by low FMRP but by the excessive amount of messenger RNA that includes the long CGG repeat (figure 5.3).

Tassone's work provided a hypothesis for why FXTAS occurs in premutation carriers, but not in people with the full mutation. FXTAS is likely to be caused by a "toxic gain of function" of RNA in carriers of the premutation form of the gene. To understand that what is meant by a *gain* of function, we need to go back to the central dogma, the model for plain-vanilla

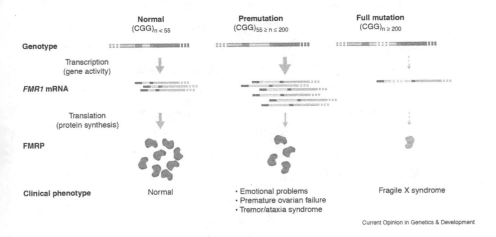

Current Opinion in Genetics & Development

FIGURE 5.3 This figure illustrates the relationship between RNA, protein, and outcome in the typical, premutation, and full mutation individual. The typical person has fewer than 45 CGG repeats. The individual with a premutation has between 55 and 200 CGG repeats. The level of mRNA is increased, causing the RNA toxicity that may culminate in FXTAS and FXPOI. FMRP, the protein, may be slightly decreased. In the full mutation, with over 200 CGG repeats, methyl groups (represented by breaks in the gene) block transcription. No mRNA can be produced: thus no FMRP can be produced, causing fragile X syndrome.

From Robert F. Berman, Ronald A.M. Buijsen, Karen Usdin, Elizabeth Pintado, Frank Kooy, Dalyir Pretto, Isaac N. Pessah, et al., "Mouse Models of the Fragile X Premutation and Fragile X–Associated Tremor/Ataxia Syndrome," *Journal of Neurodevelopmental Disorders* 6, no. 1 (2014): 25.

inherited diseases. To put it as simply as possible, according to the central dogma, mutation-carrying DNA is copied into RNA, which produces abnormal proteins. The abnormal proteins result in disease. Typically, the abnormal proteins cause a *loss* of function.

In the case of the premutation, too much mRNA with a long CGG repeat can be toxic to the cell. The excess RNA can trap other proteins that are vital to the function of the cell. And that unusual RNA, with its long repeats, can lead to the creation of small proteins that are not typically produced in a cell. In premutation carriers, brain cells called neurons and astrocytes may die early, and the tiny organelles that supply these cells with energy, mitochondria, may not function normally. When *excess* RNA and its abnormal function and products poison cells, it is known as a "toxic gain of function" of RNA. Premutation carrier conditions like FXTAS are not just a "lite" form of full mutation fragile X syndrome. Toxic RNA in carriers has its own mechanisms for destroying nerve cells.

Now that FXTAS was making itself known as a clinical entity and a worthy hypothesis as to its cause was coming together, the lab waited for a brain to examine. When Clay passed away in Colorado, Louise went with Flora Tassone and a neuropathologist, Claudia Greco, to retrieve the brain. I asked Louise why she bothered. "My job was to honor the brain," Louise explained.

Back in the lab, Greco dissected it. To her amazement, its cells were riddled with inclusion bodies, which occur when "proteins pile on like a scrum in rugby," according to Paul Hagerman.[15] They are nonspecific, meaning they are present in cells in many diseases, including Huntington's chorea, myotonic dystrophy, and other inherited movement disorders. Why they are there is unclear, but their presence is a sign that the cell is in trouble. Greco showed that in the FXTAS brain, they consisted of *FMR1* mRNA and more than twenty proteins.[16] This was RNA toxicity.

A later hypothesis, and likely both are true, was that of *repeat-associated non-AUG (RAN) translation*. In RAN translation, snippets of toxic RNA are translated into nonfunctional strings of amino acids, which are also poisonous to the nerve cell.[17] The strings can form a protein, FMRpolyG,[18] which is similar to the substance used by spiders to build webs.[19] As you might expect, it is sticky and stretchy, and it is not conducive to the healthy function of the cell.

Toxic RNA in premutation carriers particularly damages the brain, the nervous system, and the ovaries. FXTAS is something of a worst-case scenario for older carriers. The movement symptoms can be incapacitating, and as the clinicians were beginning to understand, the effects on personality and cognition can be even more devastating to the carrier and his or her family.

THE POWER OF A CASE SERIES

It took five neurologists and a case series—a small group of case presentations published together, often to call attention to a new disease—to diagnose Calvin. His wife, Vivian, who now runs an organization that provides support for caregivers, told me how it came about.[20]

Cal and Vivian met at work in Cal's Baltimore office in 1991. Cal was a prolific science writer with an entrepreneurial flair.

He founded a career coaching company that hosted classes and tutorials for scientists who wanted to write for the general public, and an intellectual society, Science Writers International. The Society held an annual international conference, and Cal and Vivian met when he hired her to assist him with organizing it and to produce written materials for the conference. When Vivian and Cal were married in 1999, he was sixty-four and full of energy.

The first time he fell was on their honeymoon.

In retrospect, Vivian had noticed a few things before they got married. Occasionally Cal would become unreasonably angry about something unimportant, and although he was generally a warm and passionate person, at times he would seem to withdraw into himself. His house was a mess. He said he would clean things up when she moved in, but he never did, and Vivian wondered why he was so careless about it. He did not seem concerned with pleasing her.

Soon after they got married, Cal began "freezing" while walking, which is often a symptom of Parkinson's disease. He would suddenly freeze, unable take a step forward or break out of his stiff posture. A neurologist conceded that Cal was stiff, but he had no tremor. Another neurologist suggested a trial of medications for Parkinson's disease, but they didn't do anything for Cal. He and Vivian sought another opinion at a large specialty care medical center, where Cal had an MRI. The neurologist there suggested physical therapy. Cal went to physical therapy for a time, but he stopped paying the bill, unbeknownst to Vivian, and the therapy was terminated.

Though Cal continued working, he became increasingly indifferent toward his former life's work. He stopped staying on top of the needs of the scientists, teachers, and writers who worked for him, and bills went unpaid. By this time Vivian was running the annual international conference herself. At Cal's last conference, in Phoenix, he slept, froze, and fell so much that the other writers could see something was wrong and inquired anxiously about his health.

Vivian told Cal he needed to retire, but he did not understand why. She decided to get another job, which he thought was disloyal. Their marriage in jeopardy, they went to counseling, but he couldn't really participate or get anything out of it. They went to a marriage encounter weekend, and while Vivian wrote letters to Cal in her journal, Cal napped.

Cal lost money in a scam. Vivian took over their finances. In 2004, Vivian brought him to yet another neurologist, their fifth. Vivian had Cal's brain MRI sent along before the visit.

This visit was different. The neurologist had just come across the biggest case series ever published about FXTAS—the twenty-six cases collected in California by Sébastien Jacquemont and Louise Gane—which detailed symptoms and MRI findings.

The first question the doctor asked was if there was any intellectual disability in the family. There was. Cal's grandson by his previous wife had fragile X syndrome. Cal and Vivian had known this all along, of course, but it never seemed worth mentioning, and no other doctor had ever asked. Two months later, a genetic test confirmed that Cal was a carrier with 121 CGG repeats. Vivian found the case series online and got in touch with Randi, as everyone does, eventually, if they are interested in FXTAS. Louise told me that Vivian might be the angriest person she had ever met.

Though Vivian had been well aware that Cal's behavior was off, she believed the hard-won diagnosis of FXTAS accounted only for his movement disorder. She believed that Cal's disorganization and carelessness had probably always been there, but she had been too in love or too "deluded" to notice. As to his apparent indifference to her, Vivian's understanding was that Cal did not love her. "I just thought he didn't care about me," she told me. No wonder she was angry.

EXECUTIVE DYSFUNCTION

What Vivian was seeing was not lovelessness, but what neuropsychiatrists call *executive dysfunction*,[21] also known as dysexecutive syndrome. As Jim Grigsby and colleagues write, "Dysexecutive syndromes are characterized by specific kinds of behavioral pathology. These include distractibility, impulsive behavior that is irrelevant or inappropriate in a given situation, perseveration, apathy, and failure to undertake purposeful activity, all of which reflect varying degrees and types of dissociation between volition and action." Put simply, we need executive function to think ahead, establish goals, and work toward them, all the while checking on our own progress, ensuring that we stay on task. Research has linked executive dysfunction with a number of psychiatric disorders, including most prominently ADHD, but also with anxiety disorders, major depressive disorder, and types of dementia (including Alzheimer's and Lewy body dementia).[22] The dementia that accompanies FXTAS is a dysexecutive syndrome.[23]

The core deficit in executive dysfunction—the "dissociation between volition and action"—has to do with mental and behavioral flexibility and the capacity to let fresh thinking take over from habit when necessary. If someone is driving to work and sees that a bridge has closed, she could decide to take an alternate route, but in the case of impaired executive function, she might give up and return home, or worse, keep driving.[24] The desire to get to work (volition) and the action undertaken to get there (driving) no longer go together in the usual way in light of new information (the bridge being out).

It was a failure of executive function that caused Cal's business to fail and his marriage to crumble. First, the career that had meant so much to Cal ceased to be important to him. He could no longer follow through with complex tasks, like organizing conferences, and was oblivious to his impairment. Later, with regard to Vivian, he was apathetic toward her and clueless about her needs. I am quite sure he loved her, but was unable focus on her, attend to her, and move from a state of loving her to actions that communicated his feelings.

About 50 percent of carrier males will develop some symptoms and signs of FXTAS by the time they are seventy, and 75 percent by the time they are eighty.[25] Only a tiny minority are as badly affected as Dave or Cal. The more CGG repeats a man has, the more likely he is to develop FXTAS. Women are much less likely to develop FXTAS, since their second, unaffected X chromosome is protective. At first, it was believed that FXTAS was a disease of men, just as at one time fragile X syndrome was thought to affect boys and men only. Unfortunately, it turns out that some carrier women do develop FXTAS (as we saw with Patricia in chapter 1), at a rate from 8 to 16 percent.[26]

FRUIT FLIES AND EMPATHY

The story of FXTAS strikes me as the story of what can happen in science when women listen to each other, but genetic counselors' empathic listening and pediatricians' intuition don't cut much ice in academic medicine. Fruit flies do.

About four years passed between Randi's first FXTAS case report and Sébastien Jacquemont's case series in the *Journal of the American Medical Association*, which was accompanied by a press release that brought widespread attention to FXTAS for the first time. Stephen Warren, professor of human genetics at Emory and editor of a prominent medical genetics journal, had rejected the Hagermans' earliest paper. A distinguished geneticist who has devoted a long career to fragile X genetics, who named the fragile X mental retardation protein and identified the gene that produces it, Warren told me, "Randi and Paul, I give them a lot of credit for pushing FXTAS, because at meetings, it seemed like something crazy."[27]

For a basic scientist like Steve Warren, FXTAS could not be connected definitively to the fragile X carrier state without a fruit fly model. Fruit flies, known by their scientific name,

Drosophila melanogaster, have been at the heart of genetic research since its earliest days. As anyone who has ever brought a banana into her home has seen, fruit flies are hardy. They breed rapidly. Their DNA is easily manipulated, and mutated progeny can be created quickly.

"We reasoned to replicate it in *Drosophila*," Warren remembered. Peng Jin and others in Warren's lab were able to use enzymes to cut out CGG repeats and splice them into fly DNA.[28] When a fly's DNA was altered in this way, it would show signs of neurodegeneration—the fruit fly version of FXTAS. For Warren and his coworkers, this was real science. Their work gave FXTAS scientific legitimacy.

Brain MRIs helped too. Once the grandfathers had had their brains examined, both before and after death, technology could confirm what was now obvious clinically: FXTAS brains *were* different. In addition to the presence of inclusion bodies, which could be detected only on autopsy, people with FXTAS had changes in their brains' white matter that were demonstrable on MRI, and they had a unique finding, not always, but usually present, called the "MCP sign." MCP stands for "middle cerebellar peduncle," which lights up on MRI in studies of patients with FXTAS and is easily recognizable to trained neuroradiologists.

According to Randi Hagerman, this last finding above all led neurologists to embrace the new "hard" neurologic disorder. Perhaps even more important for Randi, the acceptance of FXTAS opened the door to the acceptance of something in which very few people in the field believed: other, "softer" carrier symptoms, such as learning disabilities and phobias.

"General practitioners pooh-poohed these problems," she recalled, "but you can't ignore someone who is tremoring and deteriorating."

TREATMENT

Louise Gane argues that the mere act of noticing and naming symptoms breeds acceptance and healthier coping for patients. People with mysterious conditions—which might be said to include not only FXTAS, but also fibromyalgia, autoimmune diseases, and even depression—need validation and care.

Patients with FXTAS are often also diagnosed with hypothyroidism, hypertension, depression, anxiety, obstructive sleep apnea, and neuropathic pain. So, for that matter, are some premutation carriers without FXTAS. Carriers, regardless of their diagnoses, will feel better if they are not in pain and are not in emotional distress, are sleeping well, and have their blood pressure controlled. Treatment of those issues will not only improve their well-being in the present, but it will also protect their cognitive function for the future.[29]

A 2020 review of the topic of treatment of FXTAS gets more granular.[30] Some medications that are already on the market may help, such as selective serotonin reuptake inhibitors (for example, sertraline or fluvoxamine) for anxiety and depression; beta-blockers, primidone, or levetiracetam for tremor; and gabapentin, pregabalin, or duloxetine for neuropathic pain. Other medications used for neurodegenerative disorders, such as memantine, "can be tried" though results are equivocal.

A few new drugs are in development, though thus far nothing has blown researchers away. Citicoline is one: it stabilizes the cell membrane and inhibits free radicals—cellular garbage that can be destructive to the cell and requires removal. Curcumin and piperine also bind to CGG repeats with as yet unknown results. The most thoroughly studied is allopregnanolone, a neurosteroid synthesized from progesterone. It acts on receptors in the brain that are associated with calming, is protective of older neurons, and may help generate new ones. There has been one open-label trial, with only six patients treated for twelve weeks with intravenous allopregnanolone. They had no improvement in their movement disorders, but some improvement in executive function, learning, and memory.

The authors conclude: "There is no cure for FXTAS and none of the drugs mentioned previously provide enough evidence for their clinical use in FXTAS." This is hardly encouraging news, but Louise found her own ways to give hope to FXTAS sufferers, for whom there was no curative treatment. For example, Louise told me that men with FXTAS often develop problems with balance. "Men being men, they do not want to give up their independence and use a cane. I had to talk them into using accommodations." Louise recalled going to a fragile X meeting on an island in Washington, waiting to catch a seaplane. She wandered into a tourist shop where she noticed sticks carved with Pacific Northwest Indian figures. "Canes!" she thought. "They were kind of sexy." From then on, when she was talking to a patient about using a cane, she'd let him know how sexy they could be to women her age. "Don't take offense," she told me, "but I could flirt."[31]

Louise, in her sixties at the time, was the same age as many of her grandfather patients and their wives. Another diagnostic clue for FXTAS was the way the men related to her—often without the inhibitions healthy men practice when interacting with a female healthcare professional. "You've got to remember I'm a hugger and we were informal, but finally, I realized if anyone was really disinhibited [which is common in dysexecutive syndromes], they were going to kiss me . . . so I could tell if they had it." Like Randi Hagerman, Louise relied on her own experience, her sense of humor, and her careful observations of her patients' behavior to draw conclusions and dispense advice.

I had wanted to meet Randi and Louise because their approach to medicine confirmed something I have long believed as a psychiatrist: that the relationship between doctor and patient contains the seed of understanding the patient's problem. FXTAS was not discovered through technical breakthroughs, but through empathy. When doctors listen closely to their patients, with enough care, they are not just being kind. They are part of a process of discovery.

Randi's intellectual engagement and Louise's capacity for closeness allowed FXTAS to appear before them as an unforeseen conundrum that could be resolved by scientific methods and reified by the appropriate use of technology. Further, I would argue that "technology" is not just limited to MRI machines and pathologists' stains. Randi's persona—funny, loud, not above a dirty joke—grabbed attention during the medical school lecture I attended. Louise's case series, little more than a thorough list of FXTAS patients and their characteristics, made all the difference in the world to Cal and

Vivian. Cal's MRI scan was useful to his neurologist, but it was the case series that captured the neurologist's attention and allowed him to use the MRI findings to make the correct diagnosis.

A new disease must not only be recognized by a few; awareness of the condition must be propagated. Randi's and Louise's *personalities* made all the difference, not just in discovering FXTAS, but also in leading other professionals to discover their own cases.

Together, Randi and Louise presented a shifting balance of charisma, strongly stated opinion, and nurturance. Randi gave instructions, but she also heard what mothers had to say, put in the time, and tolerated disagreement by patients and by staff. "The greatest gift Randi gave me was the freedom to be myself, and for patients to be themselves," Louise told me. Louise gave out hugs and tolerated disinhibited patients who kissed her back. It was a marriage that worked. Their 100 percent commitment to their patients and their families was evident, and as Louise observed, "that situation leads to finding things if they are there."

Chapter Six

ONCE MORE, WITH FEELINGS

FRAGILE X–ASSOCIATED NEUROPSYCHIATRIC DISORDERS (FXAND)

EVEN THOUGH the "TAS" in FXTAS is short for tremor and ataxia, FXTAS is not just a movement disorder. It is very much associated with cognitive and behavioral changes, as we saw in chapter 5. For Randi Hagerman and her colleagues, the widespread acknowledgement of FXTAS as a neurological disorder was meaningful in another way: it lent legitimacy to their belief that psychiatric and other disorders tended to cluster in carriers. Now that FXTAS has been embraced by the medical community, Randi has turned toward other psychological and medical conditions she finds to be associated with the premutation. She has named these phenomena FXAND (pronounced FAX-AND), which stands for *fragile X–associated neuropsychiatric disorders*.

A 2018 paper describing the conditions explains the authors' rationale: "FXTAS and FXPOI are commonly recognized, but the most common problems of premutation carriers are psychiatric. However, these psychiatric problems are not typically recognized as related to the premutation as they do not have a fragile X–associated name. Therefore, this paper describes the fragile X–associated Neuropsychiatric Disorders (FXAND), bringing recognition to these problems by naming them."[1]

In other words, not only does the paper *propose* that psychiatric disorders are central to the lives of many premutation carriers, but it also *advocates* for their recognition. It presents not only an observation but also an argument: that psychiatric symptoms are inherent to the carrier state, and belong, with full mutation fragile X syndrome, FXPOI, and FXTAS, to one of *four* fragile X–associated groups of disorders. "Neuropsychiatric disorders are the most common problems associated with the premutation, and they affect approximately 50% of individuals with 55 to 200 CGG repeats in the *FMR1* gene," the paper states. That observation is reified into the diagnosis, FXAND.

ADVOCACY AND BIAS

Many clinicians in the field, early on, had felt that the research that had established FXTAS was contaminated by bias; and many feel that the FXAND concept is contaminated by bias as well.[2] Bias in scientific research is so great a concern among scientists that it is a subject of research itself.[3]

There are many types of bias in research, and these include *selection bias* and *confirmation bias*. Selection bias implies that the group of patients studied in Randi's lab could be different from the general population of premutation carriers, and this is likely to be true. Randi's patients tend to be identified as carriers when they have full mutation children, which implies that they have premutations in the higher range—in other words, more CGG repeats—and may be more adversely affected. Further, people who find their way to the MIND Institute and seek an evaluation by top experts are determined enough and well-funded enough to get the best care. Randi's patients include rabbis, jet pilots, renowned artists, physicists, and their children. As a rule, they are white and well-educated. Confirmation bias refers to our tendency to interpret new information in a way that confirms beliefs we already have. This is a particular danger for someone like Randi, who has very strong beliefs about the primacy of psychiatric disorders in premutation carriers. She might easily be persuaded that a patient's casual mention of anxiety was a full-blown anxiety disorder, because that is what she expects to find.

Finally, there is the idea of advocacy, which is not a form of bias but is a nonneutral approach to research. As Stephanie Sherman, the genetic epidemiologist, pointed out, speaking of Randi, "You see how she is, she is 24/7 for the families . . . it may be what families need to hear."[4] Physicians may need to hear it too. The FXAND paper says, "The importance of identifying the premutation as the etiology of FXAND is to treat . . . other complicating comorbidities such as hypertension, migraine headaches, thyroid dysfunction, and chronic pain that are associated with the premutation. It is also important so that providers can recommend the avoidance of toxins in the environment such as excessive use of alcohol or opioids, which can cause more CNS [central nervous system] disease." Randi recommends treatment of depression and anxiety with antidepressants, exercise, antioxidants, and cannabidiol.[5]

In other words, there are things both patients and doctors would benefit from knowing about premutation-associated disorders. The FXAND concept is a way to communicate directly with both about the importance of recognizing and treating these common and disturbing symptoms. Otherwise they are in danger of being brushed off.

But that is advocacy, not research.

THE BIG QUESTION: INTRODUCING CAROL

Carol is a patient of Randi Hagerman's to whom I have spoken on several occasions and who gave me permission to sit in with her on a two-day round of testing at the MIND Institute. Carol has probable FXTAS, and she also likely has FXAND. Her life story brings up the crux of a very important question: What part of Carol's physical, social and emotional difficulties is due to the fact that she is a premutation carrier, and what part is due to her life experience? In addition, Carol is by any measure an unusually successful individual. If she has FXAND, what sort of difference has it made in her life?

Growing up in a Chicago suburb in the 1950s, Carol was inexplicably scorned by her father, who expressed his contempt for her and his wife in one blow: "You're stupid like your mother." Everyone else could see that Carol succeeded at everything she did. "I self-medicated by overachievement," she now says tartly. She has a clear memory of walking outside at the age of three or four, while her parents were arguing about their finances, and asking her neighbors for change. She returned with a fistful of pennies. "I was the family social worker," she explained.[6]

Carol has retired from more careers than most of us have ever started. She has been a community college professor known for her classes on feminism; a social worker with a thriving practice in the city of Chicago; and a self-taught expert in Cesarean deliveries, whose "rap sessions" in the late 1970s helped doctors and patients understand that operative delivery could be as loving and inclusive as natural birth.

Making a positive impact on countless lives helped boost her self-esteem, but it took an autopsy for her to forgive her father— *his* autopsy.

"My dad could be a real son-of-a-bitch," recalled Carol. "He could be very cruel to my mother. He *always* called us stupid." When Carol won a piano scholarship, he told her she wasn't talented enough to use it. Nonetheless, Carol stepped up. When she decided to become a social worker, she shunned the suburbs, preferring the challenge of advocating for newly released prisoners on the south side of Chicago in the 1970s. When she became a mother, she gave it everything she had, quitting a job she loved so she could devote herself to her baby, Amy. But after a few years as a stay-at-home mom, Carol was restless and bored and found a new cause. Her daughter had been born by Cesarean section, which Carol, who always wanted to do everything exactly right, had found disappointing and dehumanizing. But rather than blame herself for "failing" at natural childbirth, Carol became an activist. She started a nonprofit organization to provide emotional support to families undergoing Cesarean deliveries. The Cesarean Birth Council International worked with anesthesiologists, obstetricians, and pediatricians, as well as new parents. It is routine today for fathers to be in the delivery room during Cesareans, but in the 1970s it required a campaign to change obstetricians' way of thinking about surgical deliveries. Carol's work helped persuade obstetricians that it was safe to have fathers be present. Then there was the postnatal experience; at the time, mothers did not hold and care for their babies in the aftermath of a Cesarean. It was considered too dangerous. The Birth Council was part of that culture change, allowing babies to stay with their mothers after delivery. As part of her work with the Birth Council, Carol observed four hundred Cesarean births, standing on a platform, "So I could see right in!"

Being diagnosed with breast cancer did not slow her down. After her surgery, which was curative, she went back to school to study feminist theory and soon had a master's degree. Then she had a cancer recurrence. Carol believes in the mind-body connection. She thought positively and used imagery and prayer. Remarkably, her cancer disappeared. She felt she had been blessed and wanted to share her experience with women everywhere.

Carol's verve and ambition had an impact on her parenting, too. Unfortunately, her eldest, Amy, did not thrive at school. Amy was introverted and a poor student. Math was impossible. Her true goal at school was never to be noticed. Contrasting Amy with her high-achieving, full-court-press mother, counselors at school told Carol that Amy's problem was that she couldn't measure up to her mother's expectations.

It's true that few children could live up to the standards Carol set for herself, and Amy confessed privately that she did feel that Carol favored her more academically successful brother, Jason.[7] But when Amy's cousin, Ben, was diagnosed with fragile X syndrome, testing of his family members—"cascade testing," in which everyone related to the newly diagnosed child is tested—provided an explanation for Amy's difficulties. Amy had full mutation fragile X syndrome. About one-third of girls with the full mutation have normal or above normal IQs, and they get by in regular schools without drawing much notice. But most, like Amy, suffer from learning disabilities and significant social anxiety. Her brother Jason had escaped fragile X completely, inheriting his mother's normal X chromosome.

Amy's diagnosis of the full mutation made Carol an *obligate* premutation carrier, as the mother of a child with fragile X syndrome. When Carol's parents were tested to see which had passed the premutation to Carol, everyone in the family was sure it was Carol's mother; Lewis, Carol's father, had called Carol's mother stupid so many times that even *she* believed it. But the carrier was Lewis.

Still, Lewis's irrational meanness and misogyny was considered just an unfortunate part of Lewis's personality, until he developed tremor, ataxia, and other symptoms of FXTAS and became an early patient of Randi's. As he aged, he grew softer, and in the end he agreed to donate his brain to Paul Hagerman's lab upon his death. When he died, Carol insisted on being present at the autopsy, though the pathologist wondered how she could stand it, reminding her, "This is your *dad* on the table." She replied, "This is my *fragile X dad*. . . . Donating was the best thing he ever did in his life." Seeing her father's brain gently lifted from his open skull helped her understand that he had loved her as much as he could.

Though some symptoms of FXTAS—for example, tremor and ataxia—are usually not evident until carriers are in their fifties or sixties, autopsies in younger men show that in fact, men with FXTAS have detectable brain changes as early as their late twenties.[8] Looking back, Carol now understands that her father's behavior was influenced by white matter changes and inclusion bodies throughout his brain, which are characteristic of some premutation carriers who eventually develop FXTAS. His executive function was severely impaired. His poor impulse control and inability to stay on task made him lash out at his wife and two daughters, unable to tolerate their spontaneity.[9]

Donating his brain, Carol believed, was her father's way of giving his family "a sacred gift . . . and I wanted to hold that sacred space."

Six years ago, Carol retired from the community college. Seventy-two at the time of this writing, she still lives in Chicago with her husband, Bill. She spends a lot of time with her two adult children, but devotes much of her energy to her latest project, motivational speaking to cancer survivors. This is her new passion.

At the same time, Carol's health has waned. She has begun to notice the symptoms of FXTAS in herself. Physically, she has noticed a mild tremor and has recently fallen several times.

As a motivational speaker, she has addressed dozens of people at a time, but one on one, she now finds she gets tongue-tied and has difficulty explaining her reasoning. She does well when she has a title, has been identified as an expert, and can speak from a position of authority. Spontaneous conversations are more challenging.

Carol notices that even though she believes her life is easier now that she has retired, she is more likely to feel overwhelmed. Although she takes antidepressants, her mood is low much of the time. She used to fight depression by succeeding wildly at everything she did; now, she notes, "I'm not as facile at compensating."

Carol's gifts and vulnerabilities have made her aware of character traits since she was very young. She is fond of using Jung's terminology of psychological types, describing herself as introverted, intuitive, judging, and perceiving. Throughout her life she has made a conscious effort to be unlike her "fragile X dad." She contrasts herself with her father's mother, who was never warm—"obviously premutated," says Carol—and indeed, Carol's grandmother was another obligate premutation carrier, because her son was a carrier. Carol is proud that *her* grandchildren call her "Silly Nana."

But speaking with Carol, one can't help but wonder whether she might possibly share some of the traits she identifies as "premutated." There is something controlled about the way she speaks of emotionally powerful topics—for example, she repeatedly describes watching four hundred Cesarean deliveries as an achievement, rather than as a privilege, a joy, or a fearsome experience. She uses jargon, describing her son as "a genius

IQ—but very right-brained." Of course, jargon can convey a lot of information succinctly; but it can also signify a lack of empathy, both for the son whom she describes so simplistically and for the listener who may not know what she is talking about.

When Carol talks about her accomplishments, it seems possible that she has told the stories so many times that she rattles them off, rather than speaking from her lived experience. Her boundless energy floods the listener, but it may also have another, unconscious, purpose—to deflect attention from Carol's cognitive and emotional difficulties.

A BRIEF REVIEW OF THE RESEARCH LITERATURE

What *does* scientific research teach us about FXAND? "Associated Features in Females with an *FMR1* Premutation," a paper of which Randi Hagerman is the senior author, lists many of the same problems as the FXAND paper, including migraines, hypertension, fibromyalgia, problems with balance and equilibrium, autoimmune conditions (particularly Hashimoto's thyroiditis), and problems with attention, executive dysfunction, restless legs syndrome, sleep apnea, ADHD, autism spectrum disorders, anxiety, and mood disorders.[10] The paper also refers to "language dysfluencies," which include repetitive speech, excessive use of "um" and "oh," and excessive revising of prior utterances. Many papers have noted these language dysfluencies in premutation carriers.[11] They are felt to represent subtle deficits in executive function.

A study that looked at premutation men who did not meet criteria for FXTAS found instead that many had ADHD and comorbid alcohol use disorders.[12] A study of mood and anxiety in women with a premutation found that the more children with full mutation fragile X syndrome in the family, and the more behavioral issues those children had, the more likely their mother was to have an anxiety disorder.

The surprising fact that there is a curvilinear association between psychiatric symptoms and CGG repeat length is highly suggestive of a biological relationship between the premutation and these symptoms. Midrange repeats in the 60–100 range have consistently been shown to be associated with mood and anxiety disorders, while carriers with fewer than 60 or more than 100 repeats are less affected. One study measured salivary cortisol levels in mothers exposed to stressful life events.[13] Cortisol, the body's natural "stress hormone," rises in response to acute stress, but in people exposed to *chronic* stress, this response is blunted. You'd expect to see their cortisol level rise when confronted with an acute stressor, but women in this study who had midrange repeats made less cortisol when confronted with new stressors compared with those with lower or higher repeats. This suggests that their chronic stress level interfered with their ability to cope with new stressors. In other words, women with 60–100 CGG repeats may already be stressed to the max. That could increase their vulnerability to psychiatric disorders.

In "A Review of Fragile X Premutation Disorders: Expanding the Psychiatric Perspective," the authors used functional MRI studies to show that in carriers, areas of the brain that are involved in processing social relationships were less active than in normal controls. This paper also hypothesized that *FMR1* protein (FMRP) levels may be below normal in premutation carriers with repeats in the upper premutation range, causing fragile X syndrome–like features in some individuals with a large premutation.[14] There are many such papers, but nearly all of them have at least one author who is connected to the Hagerman lab. The question of bias continues to dog the concept of FXAND and Randi's research in general.

A major paper published in 2019 addresses these bias concerns by "data mining"—that is, by having a computer search an enormous anonymous health database to look for patterns that might provide relevant information. In the paper "Data-Driven Phenotype Discovery of *FMR1* Premutation Carriers in a Population-Based Sample," Arezoo Movaghar and colleagues mined the electronic health records and DNA samples of 20,000 patients enrolled in the Marshfield (Wisconsin) Clinic health-care system for associations between the *FMR1* premutation and other health conditions.[15] None of the twenty thousand participants was known to have a premutation by their doctors or by themselves. Ninety-eight premutation carriers were identified by DNA testing. Their health records were compared with those of matched controls. Bias was minimized because the carriers did not know they were carriers and were not seeking care because of their carrier status. Neither they nor their doctors could have attributed an illness to their being a carrier, because none of them knew they were carriers.

The results, the paper's senior author, Marsha Mailick, explained, were "imperfect, but significant," and "reminiscent of what Randi observed."[16] The imperfection was actually a sign of accuracy, since not all premutation carriers suffer from other conditions. The paper found, indeed, that female carriers had more anxiety disorders, especially agoraphobia, social phobia, and panic disorder. They had more reproductive problems. They had more muscle pain, malaise, and fatigue. Surprising to the researchers, they had more injuries. Significantly, not only did the carriers have a greater than expected rate of these and several other conditions, but they also had earlier onset of the conditions and more doctors' visits for each of the identified conditions. In other words, their premutation-associated conditions were more burdensome.

For men, abnormal blood chemistry was the most strongly associated condition, which was unexpected, as was respiratory disease. Mood disorders and major depressive disorder were the mental disorders most commonly associated with being a male carrier.

All in all, the paper supports the concept of fragile X-associated neuropsychiatric disorders, but also points to new associations; for example, adverse drug reactions were more frequent in carriers. However, bias is not the only reason some researchers object to the FXAND concept. "It hasn't gotten much traction," said Mailick. Unlike the case with FXTAS, there is as yet no obvious causative link between anxiety and depression and the fragile X gene. And as is clear from the preceding, only partial list of associated conditions, many conditions that are *not* neuropsychiatric are associated with *FMR1* status.

The European Fragile X Network (EFXN) took a stand against the term FXAND in a statement published on its website on February 1, 2020.[17] In particular, its members believed that lumping autoimmune disorders in with psychiatric disorders did not make sense, even if autoimmune disorders might have an impact on how people feel. More strongly, they were concerned about the use of the word "disorder," which they felt was stigmatizing, preferring the word "condition."

The EFXN proposed a hierarchy of fragile X–associated diagnoses. At the top would be FXPAC, or *fragile X premutation associated conditions*. FXPAC would include FXTAS, FXPOI, and two new categories: FXANC (*fragile X associated neuropsychiatric conditions*) and FXVAC (*fragile X various associated conditions*). The last would include fibromyalgia, chronic fatigue, autoimmune thyroid disease, and other nonpsychiatric conditions, many of which Carol has.

GENES AND EPIGENETICS

In person, Carol is petite, with close-cropped copper hair, wire-rimmed glasses, yoga pants, and a big cowl-necked sweater. She looks more like a Midwestern matron than a radical peacenik. She is deaf in one ear and speaks loudly. At her evaluation, she repeated many stories she had told me years ago over the phone, to many clinicians, word for word. She spoke of being "right-brained" and mentioned being at her father's autopsy, "holding that sacred space," half a dozen times. She brought up the four hundred Cesareans and curing her own cancer through visualization and prayer. She took pride in her accomplishments, which indeed were many, but anxiously, which could lead the listener to question whether she had true confidence in herself. One sentence she repeated several times was, "I was an introvert who learned to act like an extrovert." She corrected a doctor's pronunciation of the word "perseveration" but apologized repeatedly for the occasional difficulties she had during motor testing. I thought that captured what I perceived as her unusual blend of perfectionism and insecurity.

During her evaluation, which focused mainly on her movement disorder, Carol mentioned some psychiatric symptoms, including depression, obsessional thinking, and anxiety, especially about her daughter Amy and Amy's daughter, who also has fragile X syndrome. This was either refreshingly honest or tactless, depending on how you look at it, for Amy was right there with us. Both Carol and Amy had wanted her there. Amy's role seemed to be to supply emotional support for Carol as she went through a potentially discomfiting round of neurocognitive tests. She agreed with everything Carol said about herself, punctuating Carol's statements with "That's right," or "That's Mom," often before Carol had finished speaking. Amy's facial expression was unperturbed, but from time to time, when she sensed her mother's anxiety, she hyperventilated briefly before speaking.

Of course, any grandmother would worry about her disabled child and grandchild, but Carol made it clear that she had been suffering from anxiety and depressed mood since before either was born, despite her many achievements.

She described low self-esteem from early childhood. Her trek through the neighborhood at age three or four, collecting pennies while her parents argued, is both a testament to her initiative and the story of a vulnerable child who was terrified of what was happening to her parents and needed to make it all better. She noted the use of antidepressants since the 1980s, when her children insisted she see a psychiatrist to treat her depressed mood. ("We sure did," said Amy.) She described a dramatic panic attack at the top of Yosemite Falls. And throughout her evaluation at the MIND Institute, it was clear that Carol was terribly worried about any decline in her cognition that her examination might pick up. If she could no longer overachieve, what would her life be worth?

Throughout Carol's testing sessions, I was struck by her eagerness to please, her verbosity, and her drive to assert control over her health. For an example of the last, when she had a hysterectomy some years ago, she was awake and unsedated, at her own request. She was experiencing leg pain, behind her knee, during the movement evaluation, which she described as 9 out of 10 in severity. It had started on the flight from Chicago to Sacramento. "It could be a Baker's cyst, but I'm worried about a DVT but I'm intuitive and I don't think it's a DVT," she said in response to the evaluating physician's concern. She hadn't taken any painkillers and didn't want to put off any tests, even those that required her to walk and climb. Her mood seemed fine and she didn't strike me as anxious. But at the end of her two-day visit, when she finally met with Randi, I saw it. She was tense and inarticulate. Though she spoke at length about a trip to Iran, she didn't make sense to me. (She did to Randi, though, who has been to Iran. My impression was that Randi silently filled in gaps in the conversation so that it made sense to her, but not to an uninformed observer.)

Other concerns she brought up with Randi included chronic worry about Amy—both because Amy is financially insecure and because Amy, her husband Dean, and their daughter are all disabled—and her own poor health. She reported chronic pain basically all over her body, the history of breast cancer, autoimmune hypothyroidism, and the knee pain. She described herself as "depressed" but also "cyclothymic," meaning she also experienced periods of unusually elevated mood. She had a history of obsessional "checking." She had restless legs syndrome, frequent vertigo and falls, migraines, and pain in all her joints.

Her MRI, which Randi described to her, showed the white matter disease consistent with FXTAS, scattered throughout her brain. Nonetheless, Randi gave her a diagnosis of *probable* FXTAS—you need the MCP sign (an MRI finding) for definite FXTAS, and Carol did not have it. In response to Carol's anxiety about cognitive impairment, Randi emphasized Carol's very mild tremor and minimal decline over the preceding ten years.

Though she seemed to fit the description of FXAND, from repetitive speech to chronic anxiety and depression, something Carol said about her infancy was thought-provoking. She was a full-term baby but weighed only three pounds at birth, because she and her mother had Rh incompatibility. She required special care, and, Carol emphasized, "My mother wasn't allowed to hold me for two weeks." No wonder she wanted to hold her baby after her Cesarean delivery, to the extent that it became a passion that absorbed several years of her life. How much of Carol's character related to FXAND, and how much to such severe early infantile deprivation, perhaps followed by years of verbal abuse by her "fragile X dad?"

What happens when you take a daughter with a genetic predisposition to anxiety and mood disorders and pair her with a father who is dismissive, insulting, and just generally verbally abusive? Who himself had a genetic predisposition to anxiety and mood disorders? Who himself was brought up by a mother who was "obviously premutated," to use Carol's words? Who didn't give his daughter the "good enough" parenting that helps children grow up confident and able to tolerate life's ups and downs?[18] Perhaps what we see is someone like Carol, a woman who has devoted her entire life to pleasing and sacrificing for others, but whose self-esteem hangs by an IQ point.

This is an important fact about premutation carriers: they are raised by premutation carriers.

There are several different ways that Carol's genetic predisposition to anxiety and depression—her "nature," if you will—was influenced by events external to her own genome. Her father, as Carol described him, was an abusive parent who eventually developed FXTAS. Her father's abuse was also addressed to her mother, which presumably had an impact on *her* parenting, too. These realities might be referred to as "nurture." In addition, by chance, Carol was deprived of maternal contact in a very early formative period—her first two weeks of life—which may have had an impact on her health today, more than seventy years later. Call that deprivation of nurturance "environmental."

Though people continue to debate whether "nature or nurture," and "heredity or environment," are more influential for any given human trait, most geneticists today accept the truism that nature and nurture are so fundamentally intertwined that it does not really make sense to ask the question.[19] Carol's newborn period is an excellent example of why. Because Carol's inherited blood type differed from her mother's, the treatment that was available at the time and place that she was born required them to be separated for two weeks. Carol was deprived of contact with her mother, and her mother was deprived of contact with Carol. Carol's genetic endowment—her blood type—had a huge influence on her social environment—nurturance from her mother. And the social environment that resulted had a huge influence on Carol. Then, after Amy's Cesarean birth, when, I hypothesize, Carol was motivated to form the Cesarean Birth Council at least in part due to her wish to repair her early life experience, she went on to influence the early life experiences of innumerable other infants.

The new science of *epigenetics* gives us a mechanism that explains how the environment feeds back to our genes, altering their expression, and how our genes may then direct us to alter our environment. Common sense shows us that parenting, chance, and culture can have a huge impact on children's development, that of their descendants, and that of people they don't even know.

As David Moore writes in *The Developing Genome*, his superb introduction to epigenetics:

If Barack Obama's father had not taken advantage of a scholarship in 1959 that took him from his home in Kenya to the University of Hawaii, President Obama would probably not have acquired the multicultural perspective that, in very important ways, defines him. Similarly, it is unlikely that the president's daughters—the grandchildren of that peripatetic Kenyan—would have been students at the excellent University of Chicago Laboratory Schools, where their brain structures and functions were altered through mechanisms that allow teachers everywhere to influence their students' minds.[20]

For an example of epigenetic effects on genes, one need look no further than fragile X syndrome. Epigenetics, the reader will recall, refers to chemical modifications of the gene. In the case of fragile X syndrome, that includes the CGG repeat. Epigenetic *markers* control which genes are "on"—making proteins—and which are off. One of those markers, most often associated with turning genes "off," is the methyl group. Methyl groups are molecules that attach themselves to CGG repeat chains longer than 200, and turn off the gene that makes FMRP, the fragile X mental retardation protein, resulting in fragile X syndrome.[21] So fragile X syndrome is a disease caused by an epigenetic modification of a gene that could *otherwise* produce FMRP, because the mutation is not in the part of the gene that codes for the protein. The gene is "off" because methyl groups are attached to its overly long CGG repeat.

In fact, that is just what happened when Carol was pregnant with Amy back in the 1970s. Very early in Carol's pregnancy, before the tiny blastocyst that was to be Amy had even implanted itself into Carol's uterine lining, Carol's 103 CGG repeats expanded to more than 200 repeats in Amy's DNA. The protein-coding part of Amy's *FMR1* gene is normal, just like Carol's; but because of those extra CGG repeats, Amy's gene was methylated, and thus inactivated. She can't make FMRP with the gene she inherited from Carol, and as a result, she has fragile X syndrome. Luckily for Amy, though, she is a woman. She inherited her mother's mutated X chromosome, but she also inherited her father's normal one. Because of that, she is able to make about half the normal amount of FMRP and is relatively lightly affected. She was able to marry, have a child, and work part-time. Nonetheless, she is socially inhibited and can't do many things most of us take for granted, like make change or drive on a highway.

But epigenetic modifications don't just cause diseases. "Epigenetics refers to how genetic material is activated or deactivated—that is, expressed—in different contexts or situations," Moore writes.[22] Epigenetic modifications begin at conception. All our cells have the same genetic material; remember, we all start life when an egg is fertilized and forty-six chromosomes, of which two are sex chromosomes, find themselves together as a single cell in a new union. When that first cell divides, all of its DNA is copied and two identical cells are created. But after just a few cell divisions, the developing embryo begins to sort itself into different tissues with different functions. Since every cell in our bodies contains DNA that is a copy of the first, how can we have different organs like eyes and hearts? The answer is that epigenetic modifications affect which genes are *expressed*, or are permitted to act as a template for a specific protein, at which time and place. Our cells differentiate into different types based on which proteins they create at any given time.

Epigenetics involves changes in gene *function* that are not due to the production of abnormal proteins. An epigenetic mechanism might explain how Carol's separation from her mother as an infant could leave her predisposed to anxiety and depression more than seventy years later. In a classic series of experiments in epigenetics and mothering, researchers exposed newborn rats to either high or low licking and grooming by their mothers. Presumably, for a baby rat, more licking and grooming is a good thing, and it functions as a model of attentive care and physical contact for human babies.[23] The baby rats that received more licking and grooming in the first week of their lives grew up to be more able to tolerate stress, and those that received less care as newborns were more stress-sensitive. Why?

Studies in rats and nonhuman primates put it directly: "During the postnatal period, withdrawal of maternal care, in the form of prolonged maternal separation or deprivation, can also have long-term consequences, particularly involving the development and reactivity of the hypothalamic-pituitary-adrenal (HPA) response to stress. Even variations in maternal care within the normal range can alter stress reactivity, fear responses, affect, cognition and social/reproductive behavior in offspring."[24]

The *hypothalamic-pituitary-adrenal axis* governs changes in the adrenal gland's production of cortisol, our natural "stress hormone."[25] Epigenetic modification of the gene for the glucocorticoid receptor, which allows the stress hormone cortisol to

bind to cells, affects stress-responsiveness by altering the availability of the receptor in different cell types. These epigenetically mediated changes in glucorticoid receptor density are
permanent; thus, Carol may still carry the weight of her mother's absence all these years later.

Humans are not identical to rats, of course, but there is significant evidence that the interaction between so-called *adverse
childhood experiences* (ACEs) and the glucocorticoid receptor is
quite similar between rats and human babies. A review of the
literature on adverse childhood experiences and related disorders concluded that enduring alterations of "stress-regulatory
circuits" in the brain could affect stress vulnerability and emotional regulation throughout a person's lifespan, and that this
was likely mediated by epigenetic modifications of the glucocorticoid receptor gene.

Particularly relevant to FXAND, the authors of the review
went on to ask (and suggest an answer to) a question:

Why do two individuals who have experienced very similar
patterns of ACE often show very different outcomes? This
may be partly due to social environmental or psychological
factors but also very likely in part at least due to genetic differences and epigenetic mechanisms. Emerging data suggest
that epigenetic mechanisms help to explain the association
between ACE and later health problems. Researchers have
focused on the way in which genetic variants and adverse
social environments can interact . . . and have shown that a
child's genotype may partly determine their level of risk and

resilience for later psychopathology following ACE including depression, bipolar disorder, and PTSD.[26]

Pervasive and enduring effects of early life stress are not limited to psychiatric disorders. Other conditions that have been associated with ACEs include neurodevelopmental delays, metabolic syndrome, cardiovascular disease, immune system dysfunction, and compromised reproductive health.[27] The British Birth Cohort followed more than seven thousand Britons born in 1958 for health consequences of childhood adversity, and it showed that ACEs were associated with numerous biomarkers of inflammation, which, along with ACE-associated lifestyle choices like smoking and drinking, may contribute to such disorders.

Many painful conditions have been linked to ACEs, though investigators found this was mediated by anxiety and depression.[28] Carol has many pain-related conditions including chronic joint pain, musculoskeletal pain, and migraines.[29] Of course, Carol's adverse childhood experiences include not just her separation from her mother, but also chronic verbal abuse by her father and witnessing her father's abuse of her mother. Previous research has shown that exposure to parental verbal aggression is associated with depression, anxiety, dissociation, and drug use in an enduring manner. Verbal aggression's effects have been shown to be as significant for these psychiatric symptoms as sexual abuse and domestic violence.[30]

Another research group found that verbal abuse was associated with white matter abnormalities on brain MRIs. The investigators concluded that "the brain is chiseled in precise ways by exposure to adverse early experience."[31]

OLD SCRIPTS

Zooming out a bit from Carol, let's look at her "fragile X dad," Lewis. He had FXTAS, which as we know is associated with executive dysfunction.

Research has shown that parents with poor executive functioning may have difficulty regulating their emotions and may struggle to plan, evaluate, and modulate their parenting behavior. They are challenged by the negative feelings that inevitably arise during childrearing, and they are at risk of engaging in harsh and abusive parenting tactics.

Perhaps especially relevant for Lewis, with his "obviously premutated" and "never warm" mother, investigators have linked the care children receive in childhood with the kind of care they give to their own children. "That is, parents who experienced more negative early rearing environments tend to evince more executive functioning problems," wrote the authors of a paper on executive functioning and abuse perpetration. Without the cognitive flexibility implied by adequate executive function, "risk-potentiating beliefs/schemas may automatically influence parents' cognitions and behaviors, and research suggests that the influence of such automatic processes may be especially pronounced when working memory is poor."[32]

In other words, "You're stupid like your mother" may be a knee-jerk statement blurted by a parent who has lost the capacity for truly spontaneous responses to circumstance and relies on old scripts—rather like Carol does at times.

What about Carol's parenting? Is her description of Jason as "a genius IQ—but very right-brained" an expression of maternal pride or compensation for poor working memory? Were Carol's "unrealistic expectations" for Amy as a child influenced by cognitive inflexibility, causing her to be unable to accept Amy as she really was?

I had actually met Carol's daughter, Amy, and Amy's husband, Dean, three years before, at an earlier visit to the MIND Institute.[33] I had spoken to Carol, but only on the phone, and Amy, who lives in Northern California not far from the MIND Institute, was kind enough to come to Sacramento to talk with me about being a woman with full mutation fragile X syndrome and raising a little girl who has the full mutation as well.

Amy tried to explain the way her thinking was different from that of typical kids. She remembered being given a set of blocks in grade school math, which represented numbers. Each block was a different length and represented a different number, and each was a different color. She can still remember her teacher yelling at her, "These are *numbers*, it's right in front of you," and thinking, "These are blocks."

Louise Gane, the genetic counselor, was not surprised by the teacher's lack of insight and frustration with Amy's difficulty, explaining, "When you have a woman with fragile X they will give you the verbal and facial cues that you think they're with you, but nine times out of ten they're not."[34]

Amy still has difficulty with abstract concepts and says she needs things to be concrete in order to understand them. "I need to touch things, feel them." She needs help shopping. She says despite having grown into a woman with a child and a part-time job, she still has very low self-esteem related to her school failure.

Those early school years, before her diagnosis with fragile X, were hard on Amy. And it was not just because of one insensitive math teacher. She described Carol as "hard-ass," lending some credence to her guidance counselor's assertion that one of Amy's problems was that she couldn't live up to her mother's expectations. Amy knows that Lewis was "hard-ass" toward Carol too, but by the time *she* was growing up, Lewis had mellowed with age, and like many grandparents, he was gentler than he had been with his own children. Amy told me she had once been angry at Carol for her unforgiving stance. But based on my observations of Amy and Carol, all is forgiven between them, and between Carol and Lewis as well.

WHO IS CAROL?

So who is Carol? Does she have fragile X–associated neuropsychiatric disorders (FXAND), or fragile X associated neuropsychiatric conditions (FXANC), or fragile X various associated conditions (FXVAC)? Does she even have FXTAS? What makes her who she is? These questions may be unanswerable, but what we do see is that Carol's chronic illnesses and psychological distress are in some way a product of the interplay between her genetic predisposition for such conditions and her father's predisposition for such conditions, with of course, her mother's contribution and a helping of happenstance. Top that off with the chronic stress of having a child and a grandchild with fragile X syndrome, and coping with multiple medical problems, perhaps with a paucity of the glucocorticoid receptors (which bind to the stress hormone cortisol) we all need to manage acute and chronic stressors. Finally, Carol is aging, and she can feel herself losing her edge.

These are profoundly affecting experiences, whether considered genetically, epigenetically, psychologically, or physically. And of course, Carol has a personality. With all their complexity, it is really not possible to separate these components.

Carol's case illustrates the difficulty of trying to understand the roots of a person's emotions and behavior. But just now, in Randi Hagerman's office, she was rolling up her sleeve for a skin biopsy to contribute some of her DNA to the Hagerman lab. Carol is a lifelong giver, an altruist, a problem-solver. She may have self-medicated by overachievement, as she says, but she has also cared for herself by giving wholeheartedly to others. That character trait overwhelms all the rest.

Chapter Seven

WHAT ARE FRAGILE EGGS?

TO TEST OR NOT TO TEST

SUZANNE IS a journalist in New York City who has always had access to top doctors and thoughtful, respectfully delivered medical care. In her first trimester of her first pregnancy, in 2007, like most Jewish women of Eastern European descent in the United States, Suzanne was tested to see if she carried the genes for a group of dreaded genetic diseases common to Ashkenazi Jews: Tay-Sachs, cystic fibrosis, thalassemias, and a few rarities she had never heard of. The blood test is known as the "Ashkenazi panel." Weeks went by, and Suzanne assumed all was well. When she was nearly in her third trimester, however, her obstetrician called her into the office with a piece of disturbing news: Suzanne was a carrier of fragile X syndrome.[1]

Suzanne's first thought was that her pregnancy was disintegrating. Stunned, she asked, "What are fragile eggs?"[2] The obstetrician gently corrected her, and explained that fragile X syndrome is an inherited intellectual disability—a syndrome of physical defects and developmental delay. Suzanne's X chromosome, one of two paired chromosomes that determine sex, had a minor mutation that had been identified through screening. But the minor mutation—the fragile X premutation—had the potential to expand, causing fragile X syndrome in her unborn baby.

It takes time to absorb news like that. But unfortunately, for reasons that remain unclear today, the fragile X test results did not become available in a timely manner. For Suzanne and her husband, the idea of raising a handicapped child was terrifying; that was why they had had all those tests in the first place. But despite her chops as a reporter and her need to manage her growing panic through research, Suzanne found no accessible literature about fragile X other than a few textbooks and a couple of parent memoirs. Although the condition is genetic, no one in Suzanne's family had ever had an intellectually disabled child. The information vacuum added to Suzanne's sense of impending catastrophe.

At twenty-three weeks pregnant, Suzanne already knew the sex of her baby, had chosen her name, and loved her as her child. The idea of termination was terribly disturbing, though she and her husband had no doubt that they would do it if their baby had fragile X syndrome. And Suzanne was on a very tight deadline. Because her test results had come so late, there was little time left to legally terminate her pregnancy.

At a hurriedly scheduled consultation, a genetic counselor admitted that she couldn't be sure what the fragile X premutation meant for Suzanne and her baby. Amniocentesis could tell Suzanne and her husband whether or not their baby would be born with fragile X syndrome—the baby *might* have inherited Suzanne's normal X chromosome—but it could not predict how badly the baby would be affected if the baby inherited the mutated X. Even if the baby *had* inherited the mutated X, Suzanne was having a girl. Some girls with fragile X syndrome are so mildly affected that they are never diagnosed, while others are so impaired by autism or severe intellectual disability that they cannot live at home.

Suzanne and her husband had already made peace with the fact that they would not want to raise a severely disabled child. But beyond the question of just how disabled a fragile X girl might be, there was Suzanne's premutation to think about. Like nearly everyone, including doctors they knew socially, Suzanne and her husband had never heard that word before. They knew only that there was something wrong with Suzanne, a genetic condition that had something to do with her brain, and that she had inherited it from one of her parents. Which one? What did that mean for her parents? What would happen to them all? As the genetic counseling session wound down, another scenario troubled Suzanne—perhaps her baby would be perfectly normal, but Suzanne herself would suffer the effects of the premutation and be unable to raise her.

Suzanne left the genetic counseling session feeling more frantic than ever. She had learned little about fragile X syndrome and felt the counselor was vague and unhelpful. Suzanne couldn't help being focused on dates: at twenty-three weeks, she was told, amniocentesis presented higher than the usual risks to her and to the fetus, and she had just one week left to terminate legally in New York State. If the amniocentesis results were not available until twenty-four weeks, she could get an abortion only in Colorado. As she recalled the conversation she had had with the high-risk obstetrician who performed her amniocentesis, Suzanne remembered the doctor's use of the word "intolerable": only if the risk of having a child with fragile X syndrome was "intolerable" to her and her husband would amniocentesis be justified.

Suzanne told me about her prenatal experience over a drink in a busy cafe—the kind of overcrowded Manhattan bar that allows for intimate talk precisely because so many people are buzzing around. As she shared her story with me, pausing from time to time to collect herself, it was clear that she was describing the most difficult weeks of her life.

Suzanne is small, with long brown hair going gray, which she lets surround her face in a messy way that is appealing and expresses a certain willfulness, as if to say, it's my hair and I'll brush it when I feel like it! She had pulled on a sweater dress and joked that she is entering the "mumu" phase of her life, but she still looks too young to be the mother of a twelve-year-old.

As we drank wine together, Suzanne told me that she had already been feeling ambivalent about being a mother and that raising a child with the potential for severe intellectual disability indeed seemed "intolerable." That Friday, Suzanne underwent amniocentesis. Over the weekend Suzanne and Sam stayed in bed, reading up on fragile X and checking out the price of flights to Colorado for a possible abortion. The results were in on Monday.

Amniocentesis revealed that Suzanne's baby had in fact inherited her abnormal X chromosome. But though Suzanne passed the mutated chromosome to the baby, thankfully, it had not expanded enough to cause fragile X syndrome. The baby would *also* be a premutation carrier, just like Suzanne.

Suzanne and Sam were terribly relieved when they learned that their daughter, Ruby, was only a premutation carrier. But after our conversation, which had reignited her curiosity about traumatic events she had preferred to forget, we decided to do a little more research into Suzanne's DNA. With her permission, I tracked down her DNA sample to a lab on Staten Island, where molecular biologist Sarah L. Nolin, an international expert in CGG repeat expansion, had interpreted it at the time. The DNA was still there, in deep freeze. Nolin—known as Sally to her friends—is a cheerful woman who told me that she herself would choose to abort a fetus that she knew was a premutation carrier.[3] Of course, she doesn't know Ruby.

Today, Ruby is a thriving sixth grader, an exquisite package of dry wit and charm, with a touch of goth—rather like her mom at that age. She may never feel the effects of her premutation, but it is possible that as few as a dozen or as many as eighty years from now, her son or her great-grandson will be born with fragile X syndrome. Ruby, or her daughter or granddaughter, may experience early menopause or infertility, or develop hard-to-treat pain syndromes like fibromyalgia or migraines.

"Why take the risk?" Sally asked.

A "RERUN"

One freezing cold morning, Suzanne, Sam, and I got into their car and drove over the Verrazzano-Narrows Bridge to Staten Island and the Institute for Basic Research, where Sally Nolin has worked for most of her career.

I was expecting a run-down old institution, but the building had an all-stone façade and long windows, rather like a modern architect-designed home in the Hudson Valley. Sally met us with another doctor who will be assuming her responsibilities when she retires. She is a thin woman of, at this writing, about seventy, wearing a cardigan and glasses, with short iron-to-gray hair, mostly still dark. She took us to a large "meeting room," and we sat around a table. She had pulled out several papers to give Sam and Suzanne and had also "rerun" Suzanne's DNA, which she had defrosted. Suzanne had 62 CGG repeats.

The following table illustrates how premutation expansions lead to the full mutation by CGG repeat size in a group of subjects. Notice that in women with under 55 CGG repeats, there are no children with the full mutation. The risk of having a child with the full mutation increases with CGG repeat size. For example, 81 percent of women with a CGG repeat size of 85–90 had a child with a full mutation.

Suzanne and Sam's impression after meeting with the genetic counselor had been that they had close to a 50 percent chance of having fragile X child. Basically, if the child inherited the mutated X, they believed she would most likely have fragile X syndrome. Sam noted the discrepancy on one of Sally's papers (which showed a risk of about 2 percent with Suzanne's repeat

TABLE 7.1 Full mutation expansions by maternal repeat size

Maternal repeat size	No. full mutation/ total transmissions	%
45–49	0/98	0
50–54	0/102	0
55–59	1/197	0.5
60–64	2/115	1.7
65–69	6/85	7
70–74	18/84	21
75–79	47/99	47
80–84	60/96	62
85–90	34/42	81
Total	168/918	18

From Sarah L. Nolin, Anne Glicksman, Nicole Ersalesi, Carl Dobkin, W. Ted Brown, Ru Cao, Eliot Blatt, et al., "Fragile X Full Mutation Expansions Are Inhibited by One or More AGG Interruptions in Premutation Carriers," *Genetics in Medicine* 17 (2015): 358–64

number) and remarked how different their experience would have been had they known this. Sally said, yes, the total risk is small for most women who screen positive because they are low-positives.

Sally gave Suzanne an illustration that showed a representation of her DNA. She had 9 CGG repeats, then one "AGG interruption" then 52 CGG repeats with no interruption. These numbers were meaningful.

It has long been established that the likelihood of a premutation's expanding to a full mutation increases with CGG repeat number. The premutation has been defined as a CGG repeat number greater than 55 and less than 200 because 200 CGG repeats causes fragile X syndrome, while 56 CGG repeats is the lowest number of repeats ever known to expand to above 200 in one generation.[4] Mothers with 62 repeats, as Sam noticed, have a low risk of expansion to a full mutation in one generation. However, Suzanne's premutation *did* expand, to 64 repeats in Ruby. So Ruby's risk of having a full mutation child is just a little bit higher.

Researchers are beginning to understand why some premutations expand and others don't. It has to do with what is known as an *AGG interruption*. As CGG represents the triplet of DNA bases cytosine, guanine, and guanine, AGG represents adenine, guanine, and guanine. The AGG interruption interrupts the run of CGG repeats and confers greater stability, like an anchor point.[5] The more AGG interruptions one has, the less likely one's CGG repeat number is to expand.[6]

An average, nonpremutation carrier might have a total of 30 repeats, in a pattern of 9 CGGs followed by an AGG, then another 9 CGGs followed by an AGG, and then another 9 CGGs followed by an AGG. Contrast that with Suzanne's DNA. Her CGG repeats started off as usual—just 9 followed by an AGG—but then she had 52 uninterrupted CGGs. The longer the run of uninterrupted CGGs, the greater the risk of expansion.[7]

Table 7.2 shows the same group of women as in table 7.1, now sorted by CGG repeat size and number of AGG interruptions.

TABLE 7.2 Unstable transmissions and full mutation expansions sorted by repeat size and number of AGGs

Maternal repeat size	No. AGGs	Total transmissions	Unstable transmissions*	%	No. full mutations	%
45–49	0	5	4	80	0	0
	1	32	6	19	0	0
	2	57	3	5	0	0
	3	3	0	0	0	0
	4	1	0	0	0	0
50–54	0	9	9	100	0	0
	1	49	11	22	0	0
	2	41	5	12	0	0
	3	2	0	0	0	0
	4	1	0	0	0	0
55–59	0	30	29	97	1	3
	1	95	50	53	0	0
	2	64	6	9	0	0
	3	8	0	0	0	0
60–64	0	37	36	97	2	5
	1	39	33	85	0	0
	2	38	20	53	0	0
	3	1	1	100	0	0

(continued)

TABLE 7.2 Unstable transmissions and full mutation expansions sorted by repeat size and number of AGGs (continued)

Maternal repeat size	No. AGGs	Total transmissions	Unstable transmissions*	%	No. full mutations	%
65–69	0	35	35	100	6	17
	1	28	25	89	0	0
	2	20	14	70	0	0
	3	2	0	0	0	0
70–74	0	29	29	100	15	52
	1	41	40	98	3	7
	2	14	13	93	0	0
75–79	0	43	43	100	32	73
	1	42	42	100	14	33
	2	14	14	100	1	7
80–84	0	31	31	100	27	87
	1	45	45	100	30	67
	2	20	20	100	3	15
85–90	0	8	8	100	7	88
	1	30	30	100	25	83
	2	4	4	100	2	50

*A change of one or more repeats.

From Sarah L. Nolin, Anne Glicksman, Nicole Ersalesi, Carl Dobkin, W. Ted Brown, Ru Cao, Eliot Blatt, et al., "Fragile X Full Mutation Expansions Are Inhibited by One or More AGG Interruptions in Premutation Carriers," *Genetics in Medicine 17* (2015): 358–64.

An "unstable transmission" refers to a change of one or more repeats. In the group of women with 60–64 repeats, for example, 97 percent of those with no AGG interruptions had an unstable transmission, while only 53 percent of those with two AGG interruptions had an unstable transmission.

In fact, Nolin and other researchers have proposed a possible explanation for how a normal *FMR1* gene might become an unstable premutation by *contraction*. At times, especially when the gene is passed from father to daughter, the repeat contracts—in other words, gets shorter—and at this time it may lose an AGG and its stabilizing properties. With fewer AGGs, the risk of CGG expansion rises.[8] For example, suppose a man with a premutation of 66 CGG repeats and two AGG interruptions passed a premutation to his daughter, and instead of expanding, the premutation contracted, taking an AGG interruption with it. The daughter could inherit a premutation of 59 repeats, but only one AGG interruption. Without the benefit of that second AGG interruption, her 59 repeats would actually be *more* likely to expand, let's say to 75 repeats. A person who inherited 75 repeats would be more likely to give birth to a child with fragile X syndrome.

Sally oriented Suzanne and Sam to the diagrams and papers she had brought along and to Suzanne's results. Suzanne remarked that everyone in her family of origin (i.e., parents and cousins) knew about Suzanne's status, and no one had said a word about being tested themselves. Sally sympathized with the typical family's unwillingness to see themselves as implicated in any disorders. She did advise that when Ruby is a teenager, perhaps she should begin having FSH/LH levels done every few years because if she has a tendency to experience early menopause, she might want to bear her children early, and she would certainly want hormone replacement. Sally also said that women do get FXTAS and showed Suzanne a paper stating that about 16–18 percent of women do—and that's not nothing.

Ruby does know that she is a carrier of a fragile X premutation; her parents don't keep secrets from her and consider her, despite her youth, to be capable of mature thinking about her own future. Ruby has already told her parents she wants to adopt children, and her parents don't see this as a girl's fantasy but as a likely scenario for a young woman who has definite ideas about how she wants to live. Of interest, some genetic counselors and medical ethicists have expressed concern about the capacity of children to consent to being tested for adult-onset, currently unpreventable conditions like FXPOI and FXTAS. Particular attention has been paid to *BRCA* (breast cancer gene) mutations in children, and most authors have concluded that such testing privileges parental autonomy over children's autonomy, and it is not recommended for minors.[9]

One genetic counselor whose specialty is fragile X disorders has proposed the possibility of disclosing only full mutation results to parents who have opted for prenatal testing of their fetus. A full mutation fetus could be terminated or not, as the parents choose. But it would be up to their child, when he or she reached majority, to choose carrier testing for himself or herself.[10]

I think the main takeaway for Sam was that they could have worried a lot less about having a kid with fragile X syndrome.

As for Suzanne, she struck me as inappropriately unconcerned by her risk of FXTAS. Maybe she didn't really want to know.

Was Suzanne's prenatal testing experience justified? Clearly something went terribly wrong when she did not receive a worrisome result until nearly the third trimester of her pregnancy. Maybe that was just a "glitch" of which Suzanne and Sam were unfortunate victims. But there are other reasons to avoid prenatal screening as well, as noted in this editorial, which ran in the *Journal of the American Medical Association* on July 5, 2016:

> Screening for fragile X syndrome carriers (*FMR1* gene) in the absence of family history is not recommended by any professional guidelines. The CGG triplet repeats in the low premutation range . . . are fairly common but have little chance of expanding to the full mutation range in the next generation. This screening could therefore lead to unnecessary prenatal testing and subsequent labeling of the newborns (because these pregnancies are generally continued) with unpreventable adult-onset disorders (premature ovarian failure in females, tremor-ataxia-dementia syndrome in males.) Accordingly, this approach would not be consistent with ethical conventions for predictive genetic testing in children.

But, it must be said, Suzanne *did* have a family history; she just didn't know it. True, none of her family members had had fragile X syndrome; but her mother had gone through menopause at forty-three, and her father's brother had tremor, gait problems, and what could be characterized as eccentricity versus "executive dysfunction." Either of her parents could be a carrier, and one of them was. Suzanne had never thought about these symptoms, and no one had ever asked her about them.

Suzanne had most probably technically consented to fragile X testing, which is not part of the Ashkenazi panel and is not generally offered outside of large litigious urban areas like New York and San Francisco—but all she remembers is going to a lab for a blood draw. No one had sat down with her and explained the risks and benefits of testing for each of the dozens of disorders her sample was evaluated for.

The editorial continued:

> Inclusion of a disorder in routine population screening guidelines . . . typically has required that the condition 1) be of sufficient and uniform severity that most couples would be interested in prenatal diagnosis and potential pregnancy termination if the result is positive; 2) have a set of relatively frequent and well-characterized mutations such that a positive result is predictive of disease and a negative result does not give a false sense of security; and 3) be amenable to testing by a technical platform that is cost-effective, accurate, and comprehensive for the majority of the frequent mutations. Furthermore, all of the supporting data must be fully transparent and provided to both the clinician and patient.

Suzanne's experience with genetic counseling let her down in every way mentioned here. Yes, fragile X syndrome is of a severity that most couples would be interested in prenatal diagnosis and potential termination. But no, fragile X is not uniformly severe. It can be much less so in girls, and the premutation may be unremarked upon for the carrier's entire life. On the other hand, a negative result does give a false sense of security for some premutation carriers—they may develop FXTAS or FXPOI, and some premutation carriers may have learning differences and anxiety and mood disorders. Technical aspects of testing clearly went awry as Suzanne did not learn of her results until it was nearly too late to respond to them at all. And finally, there is virtually no *data* supporting *FMR1* premutation testing or not.

Amy Cronister, the genetic counselor involved in the discovery of FXPOI, spoke to that point.[11] The idea that women wouldn't want to know their own and their baby's fragile X status doesn't make sense to her, regardless of what they decide to do with the information. She notes that women test routinely because of concerns over Down syndrome, even though in her view, Down is less burdensome than fragile X syndrome, because families usually have only one child with Down syndrome, since it is mostly sporadic, and children with Down typically don't have the problems with agitation and outbursts that fragile X children do. "There are waitlists to adopt children with Down," she said, "yet women want to be tested. Why for that and not for fragile X? With fragile X, it's carriers that have held things up. A woman who is a carrier, what will she do if she has a female fetus [who might be very mildly affected] or needs follow-up care herself? We don't have enough information."

BIG DATA

One genetic testing company, Counsyl, took on that issue by funding a study of "expanded carrier screening" in a very large population, of 346,790 individuals. This study, also published in the *Journal of the American Medical Association*, pointed out that "ethnicity based testing"—the current gold standard—depends on people accurately reporting their own ethnicity, which they may not always be able to do.[12] The Counsyl study used mathematical modeling and data from more than 300,000 patients to show that fragile X mutations were more common than spinal muscular atrophy and cystic fibrosis in nearly all ethnic groups. These are conditions for which pregnant women in the United States are universally screened.

Counsyl has since changed its name to Myriad Women's Health, perhaps reflecting its new emphasis of the number of diseases screened for versus its role in counseling women on how to interpret and use test results. A newer study by Myriad addresses the cost-effectiveness of expanded carrier screening, showing that the conditions it screens for rob affected children of an average of twenty-six years of life and cost approximately $1,100,000 per affected child.[13]

It was only a matter of time before the American College of Obstetricians and Gynecologists (ACOG) altered its prenatal testing recommendations to include expanded carrier screening as a *possible* option for all women (it stopped short of *recommending* it for all women).[14] The ACOG leaves a little wiggle room in not recommending testing for fragile X in women without a family history, if they don't opt for an expanded carrier screen.

For women who *do* opt for expanded carrier screening—and Counsyl data suggest that up to 50 percent of the four million women who become pregnant per year in the United States will in the near future—they will be tested for fragile X, as Suzanne was. ACOG further suggested, to encourage fair utilization of resources and impede bias, that each ob-gyn or group practice adopt one approach that it would recommend for all patients.

BEFORE CONCEPTION

"It used to be so simple," observed high-risk obstetrician Ronald Wapner of Columbia University Medical Center in a 2019 editorial regarding screening. Those were the days when a prenatal test for Tay-Sachs disease was first discovered in the 1970s, and the most successful prenatal detection program ever devised was developed within New York's Orthodox Jewish community.[15]

The Committee for the Prevention of Jewish Disease (also known as Dor Yeshorim) was founded by a rabbi who had lost four children to Tay-Sachs disease.[16] Tay-Sachs is inherited in an autosomal recessive manner, meaning that both parents must be carriers of the disease for it to appear in their children. Carriers have no symptoms and no way to know that they are carriers unless they have genetic testing. Of their children, approximately one in four will develop Tay-Sachs, a disease that begins in infancy and usually results in death by the age of five.

Tay-Sachs represented a perfect storm for the Orthodox Jewish community in New York City. There was a large population of Orthodox Jews intermarrying, big families were encouraged, and abortion was forbidden. Fortunately for the community, religious law dictates that Jewish people have an obligation to care for their own health. Rabbi Eckstein, the father, forged relationships with doctors at Mount Sinai Hospital, partnering with its chairman of medical genetics, Dr. Robert Desnick. With the help of community leaders, they developed Dor Yeshorim, a preconception screening program that was acceptable to the community because it took into account the requirement for arranged marriages and the shame associated with being a carrier of a horrific familial disease.

When they are in high school, boys and girls approaching marriageable age are screened for Tay-Sachs carrier status, along with several other genetic diseases. The screening is anonymous, and each sample is identified by number. When a match is arranged, the couple requests evaluation of their match from Dor Yeshorim. If both members of the couple are carriers of any of the diseases on the panel, the match is called off without anyone's needing to know the reason.

The general availability of stigma-free testing has virtually eliminated Tay-Sachs from New York's Orthodox Jewish community and many other such communities worldwide. Of eligible high school students, 90 percent opt for testing. Before Dor Yeshorim was created, there were sixteen beds at the Inborn Errors of Metabolism Unit at Kingsbrook Jewish Medical Center, and a waiting list for care. In 1996, the last child with Tay-Sachs died. Since then there have been no new cases.

Expanded carrier screening is different. It was not developed with a specific community in mind, or even a specific disease. There is no consensus on what should be tested for. Of sixteen currently available commercial panels, only three diseases appear on all of them.[17] Some panels contain diseases so rare that virtually no physicians have ever heard of them—for example, Salla disease, which has been reported in a total of two hundred people of Finnish descent. The panels are created and promoted by genetic testing companies, not by individuals dedicated to the special circumstances of a specific community. Ob-gyns don't have the time or training to implement them properly.

Wapner advocates moving all prenatal carrier screening to the preconception period, as Dor Yeshorim did. As Suzanne and Sam found, pregnancy is a high-stakes setting in which to learn that one may carry a serious genetic condition. But even for those who know they are carriers prior to conception, pregnancy brings new pressures. Few women know how they will feel when they are pregnant, until they are.

ANOTHER SIDE OF PRECONCEPTION SCREENING

Consider another prenatal screening story. Melanie was actually screened before she was pregnant.[18] She had been told she had polycystic ovarian syndrome (PCOS), which was diagnosed when she was a college student, after years of irregular periods. Because her menstrual cycle continued to be unpredictable, she anticipated difficulty conceiving, and when she and her husband were ready to have children, they went to a fertility specialist for advice. He suggested they get an expanded carrier screening panel. Said Melanie, "I blindly followed his advice."[19]

At the time, Melanie was in law school. Today she is a lively, warm, new mother, touchingly honest about how much she loathed being pregnant. Back then, she was busy and distracted. She got a phone call from the genetic counselor who had ordered the expanded carrier screening panel. Already annoyed that the test had cost more than a thousand dollars, she was nonplussed when the counselor told her she was a fragile X carrier. The counselor assured her it was nothing to worry about, but she might want to have more testing when she got pregnant. "I'll probably never get pregnant anyway," Melanie remembers thinking. But after just a few months of trying to get pregnant the old-fashioned way, she did.

Now that she was pregnant, Melanie saw an obstetrician and told him about her fragile X carrier status. He suggested a meeting with another genetic counselor. Melanie had 57 CGG repeats, within the premutation range, although the risk of expansion to a full mutation in her baby was "very low," according to her genetic counselor. However, no one could assure her that the risk was zero.

Melanie had always been an anxious person and had taken medication for anxiety before pregnancy. Now pregnant, with no medication in her system, Melanie developed a crippling obsession with fragile X syndrome. She read up on it constantly, could not put the idea that she might have a baby with fragile X syndrome out of her mind, despised herself for being reluctant to have a child with an intellectual disability, and became convinced that her "bad gene" was "poisoning" her unborn child. During this crisis, she was unable to make a decision about how to move forward. She was offered CVS—chorionic villus sampling, which can be done in early pregnancy—to assess the fetus and scheduled an appointment, but then cancelled it. She was frightened of inducing a miscarriage, and she worried that since she knew she was having a girl, she might not want to terminate the pregnancy even if the baby *did* have fragile X syndrome, asking herself, "How could I terminate a baby that might only have dyslexia?" But after changing her mind about having CVS, the uncertainty remained unbearable for her. After weeks of "agony," she decided to have amniocentesis, only to cancel and reschedule three times. At her last amniocentesis appointment, she sat sobbing in the waiting room, unable to enter the procedure area, and finally went home.

Melanie consulted a psychiatrist, and after several weeks she agreed to take medication to help her feel more like herself. It did help her stabilize, and although she remained worried, she delivered a healthy child. Even after the baby was born, however, she continued to obsess about fragile X in the baby, although she was meeting her milestones and developing well. At four months, the baby was tested for fragile X. There was nothing. She had inherited Melanie's normal X chromosome.

As Melanie reflects on her experience, she believes she had the wrong obstetrician for a woman with so severe an anxiety disorder. "He would say things like, 'Oh, the risk of CVS is that only one in 500 miscarry, but if you're the one out of 500, that's not going to be comforting.'" The same OB gave her a piece of misinformation about amniocentesis, leaving her wondering, "Do these doctors even know what they are talking about?" Her genetic counselor, Erica Spiegel, became her most trusted guide.

Erica is in her thirties at this writing, and she is very knowledgeable about fragile X disorders. I have spoken with dozens
of scientists and never encountered anyone who speaks of fragile X mutations with her degree of clarity. She gave me a full
hour of her time at the busy medical center where she works in
New York City. The waiting area was crowded with couples and
stressed-out pregnant women, including one Orthodox Jewish
woman praying and rocking silently.

Erica's attitude toward genetic counseling is more matter-of-
fact than Louise Gane's. She is younger, less maternal, and
more businesslike, and this is reflected in her approach to the
patient. "I meet them where they are. I'm a sounding board."[20]
She believes most patients already know what they want to do
before they even meet with her; they just need to talk it out.

Amniocentesis was once considered a standard procedure for
women over thirty-five years of age who wished to avoid Down
syndrome, but now that noninvasive prenatal testing, also
known as cell-free DNA testing, is available, Erica's clinic
requires anyone undergoing amniocentesis or CVS to meet with
a counselor first. Noninvasive prenatal testing, commonly
known by its acronym as NIPT, allows a tube of the mother's
blood to be used to analyze the fetus's DNA. It can rule out
Down syndrome without the need to stick a needle into the
uterus or placenta, and so invasive testing is no longer considered routine at her clinic, even though the American College
of Obstetricians and Gynecologists still recommends that it be
offered to all women.

Erica likes to send her fragile X samples to Sally Nolin on
Staten Island for faster results than she can get from a genetic

testing company. Sally told Erica that with 57 CGG repeats, Melanie's risk of expansion to the full mutation was "infinitesimal" but could not be completely ruled out. There is that one case report of a woman with 56 repeats expanding to a full mutation in one generation.

Melanie was a special case for Erica because she was so anguished and unable to come to a decision about testing, let alone abortion of an affected fetus. Erica finally departed from her usual practice of neutrality and advised Melanie to have amniocentesis to put her distress to rest, but Melanie could not go through with it. Erica finds that mothers vary in how risk-averse they are with regard to invasive testing, and that many have strong, often secret beliefs about having a child with intellectual disability. With fragile X, the combination of intellectual disability and behavioral challenges is especially worrisome.

In addition, in an X-linked disorder, the woman has a tendency to blame herself, as Melanie did, believing her genes were "poisoning" her baby. In recessive genetic diseases, both parents are "responsible" for passing on the condition. One of Erica's major goals in counseling sessions is to assuage parents' guilt, regardless of the condition their fetus may have.

Another is giving the patient just the right amount of information. The inheritance of fragile X syndrome is quite complicated, as we have seen. And the likelihood, severity, and personal significance of the premutation's causing FXTAS or FXPOI in oneself or one's child is an unknown. A pregnant woman like Suzanne may be calmed by doing her own research and being given a diagnosis of the premutation in her daughter, without requiring more information. Other women might feel the need to know a great deal more about the premutation, while still others, like Melanie, might be unable to absorb anything due to her severe anxiety and guilt. For Erica, finding a balance between appropriate disclosure and information overload is part of the art of genetic counseling.[21]

Like Suzanne, Melanie used the word "intolerable" to describe how she felt about raising a child with intellectual disability. But unlike Suzanne, Melanie had not made peace with those feelings. She was deeply shamed by the idea that there was a type of child who would be unacceptable to her, and in particular, the thought that she might abort a female fetus whose worst problem might be ADHD or a learning disability was unbearable.

Melanie is certainly an example of someone who suffered profoundly because of preconception genetic testing. She can't undo that testing, but if she has another child, she plans to undertake CVS as early as possible in the hope of putting the full mutation question to rest early in pregnancy. How she will fare if her child, like Melanie herself, is a premutation carrier remains to be seen.

PATIENTS-IN-WAITING

Sociologist Gil Eyal has written about the way "precision medicine" may be expected to impact the patient in unexpected, nonbeneficial ways. "Precision medicine . . . raises the possibility that instead of preventing diagnostic odysseys, precision medicine will introduce a new type of 'therapeutic odyssey'"[22] as the newly diagnosed patient tries to figure out what to do with an unanticipated illness with no current manifestations. Suzanne and Melanie both experienced agonizing "therapeutic odysseys" as they tried to figure out what to do with incomplete information in the high-stakes setting of mid-trimester pregnancies.

Further, Eyal points out, women like Suzanne, Melanie, and even twelve-year-old Ruby have become "patients-in-waiting"— currently healthy women who may one day develop FXTAS, FXPOI, or other conditions not yet elucidated. Genes sound the alarm for events that may take place in the future, but in the present, those possibilities may seem completely irrelevant.[23] In the meantime, all carriers can do is wait and hope that they will be part of the large majority of carriers who never experience any deficits from their premutations.[24]

Chapter Eight

BORDERLANDS OF THE PREMUTATION

GRAY ZONES, LOW-NORMALS, AND ENDOPHENOTYPES

FRAGILE X syndrome—the full mutation—has been in the medical literature since the early 1940s, when it was first described by James Purdon Martin and Julia Bell, and it became known as Martin-Bell syndrome. In 1969, Herbert Lubs discovered the fragile site, and the condition was ultimately renamed fragile X syndrome. But it wasn't until the early 1990s that the whole picture of fragile X inheritance began to fall into place, when the premutation was discovered and its role in causing fragile X syndrome explained the Sherman paradox.

The Sherman paradox isn't really a paradox at all, but a description of an aspect of the inheritance of fragile X syndrome (see chapter 2). As the generations in a family descend, each generation has more members with fragile X syndrome. A man is more likely to have a grandson with fragile X than a brother who has it. This seemed paradoxical at first, since it was so unlike typical genetic diseases. But the existence and function of the unstable, expanding premutation explained it. As the premutation lengthened through generations, more and more children would be born with the full mutation. Older family members were carriers, but to all appearances they were normal.

The Sherman paradox shows us that people who *don't* have fragile X syndrome teach us as much about fragile X inheritance as people who *do* have it.

Sometimes it's looking at the edges of a problem that clarifies it. To further understand the premutation, it's necessary to look at some aspects of the premutation that may or may not be pathological. In other words, they may or may not be associated with disease.

THE PLACES IN BETWEEN

Attentive readers may have noticed something: there is a group of people whom I have left out of my discussion of CGG repeat numbers, and as it turns out, it's not a small group. These are people who don't fit into the categories "normal" (under 45 repeats), premutation (55–199 repeats), or full mutation (at least 200 repeats). These individuals, who have 45–54 repeats (some say it's 41–54 repeats) are considered to be in an intermediate or "gray zone."

The rate of *FMR1* gray zone expansions in the general population is variable, but large population studies report rates as low as 0.8 percent to as high as 3.0 percent for repeat sizes between 41 and 54.[1] That's a wide range, but even 0.8 percent of the population is a huge number of people.

The gray zone has some similarities and differences from the premutation. The most significant difference is that there has never been a known case of transmission from the gray zone to the full mutation in one generation. In fact, this is one of the reasons the upper limit of the gray zone was chosen to be 54. However, there is one case report of a family in which a grandfather was in the gray zone, his daughter had a low premutation, and her son had the full mutation.[2] In this family, it took just two generations to move from gray zone to fragile X syndrome.

AGG interruptions, which stabilize the strip of CGG repeats, also play a role in the gray zone's significance for any particular individual. Typically, only gray zone mutations with one or no AGG interruptions can expand; those with more AGG interruptions remain constant. In the case of the family just mentioned, which transitioned from gray zone in the grandfather to full mutation in the grandson, two AGG interruptions were present in the grandfather's gray zone repeat. But the AGGs were lost when the repeat passed to the mother, and without AGGs to anchor her premutation, her child inherited a full mutation.

The gray zone presents a number of clinical and scientific challenges to researchers. Most researchers now agree that 54 is the upper limit, since 56 is the lowest number of CGG repeats that has ever expanded to the full mutation in one generation. However, some researchers prefer a lower bottom limit than 45, because there have been case reports of patients with fewer repeats showing some FXTAS and FXPOI-like symptoms. Interestingly, the rising level of *FMR1* mRNA, which is felt to be responsible for FXTAS and FXPOI, begins to increase at around 39 CGG repeats.[3] So while changes at 39 repeats may not have shown up clinically in patients, in the lab they are noteworthy.

The most-studied consequence of gray zone alleles (an allele is a variant version of a gene) is the presence of parkinsonism. Neurologist Deborah Hall of Rush University Medical Center in Chicago writes, "Our group found [that] 5.5% of parkinsonism patients (n=273) overall in movement disorder clinics were *FMR1* gray zone carriers and that 12% of the female parkinsonism patients (11/98) had gray zone alleles. Clinical characteristics of the gray zone carriers included classical features of Parkinson's disease (PD), with most patients having asymmetric rest tremor, bradykinesia [slowed movements], and rigidity."[4]

Another group, based in Australia, conducted similar studies. They found a significant excess (8.2 percent) of gray zone carriers with parkinsonism compared with 5.2 percent in the control sample without parkinsonism.[5]

In Iran, a research group investigated the possible association between Parkinson's disease and *FMR1* expanded alleles, looking for both gray zone and premutation carriers. They screened 154 male Parkinson's disease patients versus healthy controls. Eleven gray zone carriers (7.14 percent) were detected among the Parkinson's group compared with just three gray zone carriers (1.57 percent) among the controls. No premutation carriers were identified.[6]

Perhaps most shocking, Deborah Hall's group found that the gray zone was associated not only with parkinsonism but with earlier death: "In examination of the demographic data in both male and female gray zone carriers, age at death was approximately 3 years earlier than in individuals who were noncarriers. Gray zone carrier men also had a lower educational level than noncarrier men by almost 2 years."[7] In addition to movement disorders, FXPOI has been reported in one gray zone carrier in Turkey.[8]

TOO FEW CGGS IS NO SAFEGUARD

A few too many CGG repeats can put a person into the gray zone range. But having too few repeats is associated with problems of its own. There is another oddity of CGG repeat length, and that is the "low-normal" repeat. A Wisconsin-based study of more than ten thousand adults found an average CGG repeat number of 30.6. Two standard deviations from the mean—roughly, below the average, but not *that* far below—was 23 CGG repeats. The researchers looked at men with 23 or fewer repeats, and at women with 23 repeats or less on both X chromosomes. They found a few surprising things.[9]

Perhaps most surprising (to me, at least) was the two and one half times higher risk of breast cancer in women with 23 or fewer CGG repeat alleles, and four times the risk of uterine cancer.

The authors noted that previous work had suggested that low CGG numbers might increase the survival of embryos carrying *BRCA1* and *BRCA2* mutations, allowing them to live long enough to develop cancer.[10]

The study further showed associations between low CGG repeat numbers and having more problems with memory and daily living in older adults, and a higher likelihood of having a child with mental illness or intellectual disability. Oddly, older women with low repeat numbers were six times as likely to need more drinks to get as tipsy as they had in their youth.

The authors concluded that tight control of CGG repeat number within a small specific range may be necessary for optimum outcomes.

A WHISPER OF AUTISM: AN ENDOPHENOTYPE

Margaret was forty-six when we spoke for hours by phone.[11] Dr. Randi Hagerman had suggested that I contact Margaret because she provided an example of the broad autism phenotype, a recently described *endophenotype* originally recognized in parents of children with autism. An endophenotype is a presentation of a condition, like autism, that is so mild that it doesn't constitute a diagnosis. It's more of a clinician's impression than a full-on disorder. So the broad autism phenotype doesn't describe a person with autism, but a person with what might be called a hint of autism.[12]

The *Harvard Mental Health Letter* explains the "endophenotype" concept very clearly, emphasizing its usefulness to scientists. "'Pheno-' means showing or appearing. The pheno-type of a disorder is its immediately observable signs and symptoms. 'Endo-' means internal or inside; an endopheno-type, also called an intermediate phenotype, refers to a charac-teristic that is not easily observed on the surface. People with a given endophenotype are more susceptible to the disorder, and that fact reveals something about the biological processes that underlie the disorder."[13]

Geneticists like endophenotypes because they are thought to reflect underlying genetic predispositions. So a mother of an autistic child might not herself be autistic, but investigation of her genome might reveal genes she has in common with her autistic child. Such a discovery can help geneticists home in on genes of interest.

Molly Losh, an autism specialist at Northwestern University in Chicago, summed up what is known about the so-called broad autism phenotype (abbreviated as the BAP):

> Converging evidence from a number of . . . studies indicates that certain personality traits and social behaviors are observed more commonly among autism relatives than con-trol relatives of individuals with Down syndrome. . . . Both family history and direct assessment studies have reported elevated rates of socially reticent, or aloof personalities among autism parents, as well as untactful behavior, and fewer high quality (i.e., emotionally reciprocal) friendships. Autism relatives have also been reported to more commonly display rigid personalities, showing relatively little interest in novelty or difficulty in adjusting to change in environment

and activities, as well as perfectionistic or overly conscientious, detail-oriented traits. Finally, anxiety-related features (e.g., anxious and hypersensitive personalities, increased rates of anxiety disorders . . . also appear more common among parents of individuals with autism. These characteristics closely correspond to the social impairments, ritualistic/repetitive, and anxious behaviors observed in autism, making them good candidates as autism intermediate phenotypes.[14]

Randi had treated Margaret's son, Joseph, for fragile X syndrome with features of autism. Over the course of the treatment, she had come to know and become quite fond of Margaret. Randi's clearest memory of Margaret is the repeated phone calls Margaret made to her during the early years after Joseph's diagnosis. Not that most mothers don't want to talk to Randi, but Margaret was particularly relentless, asking the same questions over and over, almost begging at times for reassurance that her son would be "normal."

Margaret is well-intentioned and was very helpful to me, tolerating a lengthy interview and sharing her life history unsparingly. But "untactful," "rigid," and "hypersensitive"—Molly Losh's terms—seem to me to be accurate descriptions, and I think that Margaret would acknowledge them.

She describes an isolated childhood, with depression and eating disorders as far back as she can remember. She had no friends and was bullied. Her interests were, and still are, solitary: reading, knitting, libraries. She told me, "I'm depressed, I'm not normal, I was weird in school. I would do what anyone wants if I would meet a man." That last sentence is what executive function researchers call impulsivity, and BAP researchers call "lack of tact"—a failure to inhibit a conversation-grabbing digression.[15]

Margaret was hospitalized twice as a teen with bulimia. She described driving around her hometown alone, binging and purging in the car. "I had severe depression, always, problems getting along with people, choosing bad men, in very abusive relationships, bad choices. I don't feel good about myself. Whatever I do, it doesn't work out."

Margaret's experience with fragile X began when her son Joseph was born. She found out she was a carrier when he was diagnosed, after she noticed that he was not meeting his milestones like his brother, two years older. It's apparent, speaking with Margaret, that she is very intelligent but has difficulty expressing her thoughts appropriately, which is consistent with the BAP, but also more generally with the premutation in some patients. Many researchers have shown that the cognitive profile in symptomatic premutation carriers predominantly shows executive function deficits.[16] Margaret's *behavior* from her youth to her current age is rife with executive dysfunction. But this impairment is also visible in *how* she tells a story; it's full of non sequiturs, repetitions, oversharing, and an inability to judge how she is being heard.

Remember, the role of executive function is to prioritize, plan ahead, process feedback, and stay on task. It seems that one aspect of the BAP is that it's a form of executive dysfunction applied to *language*.

Some researchers divide BAP-related language dysfluencies (a dysfluency is a small speech mistake, like saying "um") into two camps. Individuals who control conversations and are excessively verbose have a "dominating" style, which surely applies to Margaret: "overly detailed, vague, tangential, overly frank, pedantic, overly talkative, no reciprocation, topic preoccupations, and interruptions."[17] Those with a "withdrawn" style offer too little information and require much prompting.

Even female *infants* who carry a premutation, who are too young to speak, can display behavioral, gestural elements of the BAP. In one study, premutation carrier babies had fewer gestures and poorer eye gaze.[18] The authors write: "These results suggest that infants with a premutation may present with subtle developmental differences as young as 12 months of age that may be early markers of later anxiety, social deficits, or other challenges thought to be experienced by a subset of carriers."

WHY BOTHER WITH THE BAP?

About 14 percent of premutation boys meet criteria for autism spectrum disorders, and about 5 percent of girls do.[19] But as we have seen, the premutation-related *endophenotype*—the hint of autism spectrum disorders, evident from birth—may be more common than was previously appreciated. On the other hand, both Melanie and Suzanne, the pregnant women identified by screening in the previous chapter, are gregarious, outgoing, empathic, and in touch with their own feelings.

So why should anyone care about the BAP, which is not even considered a disorder, but an unusual personality style? Because the premutation carrier's susceptibility to the BAP may shed light on the cause of idiopathic autism, or autism of unknown cause. *FMR1* mutations are the most prevalent known *single-gene* cause of autism. That means that investigation of mutations involving the *FMR1* gene can help researchers learn about autism in general. When we know precisely what *FMR1* mutations do in the brain, we will understand at least one relatively common form of autism, and with luck we can extrapolate it to others.

This relationship is far from completely understood, but it seems that FMRP, the protein absent in fragile X syndrome and poorly regulated in the premutation, interacts with more than a hundred different genes that are suspected to be involved with autism.[20]

Thus, FMRP has an effect on multiple genes that may lie behind the complex, *multi-hit* genetic disorder that is autism (multi-hit means that many things have to go wrong to lead to the disorder). Abnormalities in FMRP production and in *FMR1*-associated RNA could constitute some of the many "hits" that are hypothesized to be responsible for autism of unknown cause.

STUCK IN THE MIDDLE

Much research has shown that while mild autistic features dominate in male premutation carriers, obsessive-compulsive features, or more generally anxiety, are found in female carriers.[21] (See chapter 6.) Because all premutation men pass their X chromosomes and their premutations to all of their daughters, this leads to a recurring situation in carriers: that of a young girl who is anxious and obsessional being raised by a father who is rigid, perfectionistic, and has limited interests, often of a solitary nature—in other words, a father with the BAP.

When Mara was just twenty-five, before she considered having children, she saw a gynecologist to evaluate her chronic pelvic pain. The pain was so bad that after walking around for several hours working the night shift at a cable news station, she could barely stand. While undergoing this diagnostic workup, which incidentally resulted in a diagnosis of FXPOI, she could not help noticing the way her father was changing. He had developed a tremor and was having trouble getting up from a chair. A neurologist had diagnosed him with Parkinson's disease. Now we know better: Mara's father had FXTAS.

Mara's father, Stefan, had retired from a career as a certified public accountant. His hobby was rocketry. His greatest pleasure, Mara told me, was blowing things up. As a much younger man, he was prone to road rage and did not seem to care that his reckless driving put his children in danger. He hardly played with his kids, although he would take them along on rocket launches and to hobby stores, often lecturing them on technique. He never joked and rarely laughed. When I asked Mara if she ever wondered if he was on the autism spectrum, she said she had. When I asked her if she ever wondered if *she* were on the autism spectrum, she said no: "I think it's more that I was raised to think nothing I ever did was good enough. Now I can't look anyone in the eye because I am so unsure of myself."

Forty-two at the time of this writing, Mara has been lucky enough to have two sons: Tommy, twelve, and Matt, fourteen, each of whom also carries a premutation.[22] Her boys are what Randi calls "high-level" premutation carriers, with 180 and 166 CGG repeats respectively. Unfortunately for them, that is a *double hit*. They have symptoms related to toxic RNA from their expanded CGG repeat lengths, but they also are likely to have a drop-off in FMRP levels from those of kids with smaller premutations or no mutations.[23] Often individuals with higher repeat numbers don't make a normal amount of FMRP, even though they make enough to stave off fragile X syndrome. Neither boy is intellectually disabled, but both struggle with mental health and behavioral problems. "I love my sons," Mara told me. "But this has been hell."

Tommy, the "more obviously strange" boy, according to Mara, has been diagnosed with ADHD and mood instability. He is anxious and has a phobia of pigeons. Crowds, smells, and loud sounds upset him, and he has poor coordination with difficulty writing. He is good-natured but very vigilant. "He talks all the time, runs ahead of everyone else in the group—it can be hard to take. Matt beats the shit out of him, because it drives him crazy," Mara said. Tommy takes clomipramine, an older antidepressant, for his phobia, and Intuniv and Ritalin for ADHD. He takes Abilify to stabilize his mood.

Tommy's speech is notable for several dysfluencies. He stays on a subject too long when the moment has passed, and occasionally he will talk baby talk or use the third person inappropriately. Although he has been evaluated for autism and more than one psychiatrist has told Mara that he does not meet criteria, he doesn't look people in the eye, and he talks to himself. His speech is "cluttered," with words that bunch together, and he often leaves out a letter or a word. These are examples of "pragmatic language violations"—pragmatic referring to how language is *used* in conversation. In my view, Tommy may not meet criteria for autism, but he surely meets criteria for the BAP.

Matt has been diagnosed with bipolar disorder. He had his first manic episode in sixth grade, when his pediatrician started him on Zoloft to treat his anxiety. He became sexually preoccupied, got knives out and carried them around, and beat his little brother with a rod. He told his mother, "I'm having violent thoughts but I don't want to kill anybody." Now he takes Intuniv, Ritalin, Effexor, Abilify, and Depakote, a second mood stabilizer.

The kids can be bright, curious, and loving. But, Mara says, "In the closet we have this nightmare at home. It's like being trapped in a hostile relationship. The kids can be horrible and terribly violent, and terribly mean, behind closed doors. We don't have babysitters, and my parents won't watch them."

They can be tricky, too, accusing their parents of shoving and hitting, when in fact the children were about to harm each other and needed their parents to separate them. "They don't have an off-switch and can't regulate their behavior, so they can't do horseplay," Mara explained.

Mara has been very disappointed in psychiatrists, who know next to nothing—in fact, usually absolutely nothing—about the premutation or the BAP and how they might be affecting the boys. The many psychiatrists she has taken them to generally blame her parenting and suggest parenting classes. They have told her that her expectations for child behavior are unrealistic, and that she needs to show the kids that she is in charge.

Mara admits she is angry and has to guard against feeling paranoid. At a prestigious child psychiatrist's office, as he told her she just needed to relax, she fumed as she looked at the pictures of the psychiatrist's kids in their sailing uniforms. "He didn't get it. I brought fragile X literature—he just wasn't interested."

Mara told me that deep down, she can't accept her kids' having so many problems. The boys stay indoors most of the time and don't run around with the neighborhood crew, skateboarding or playing soccer. She knows it doesn't help, but when she compares her family to her sister's "perfect" one, it hurts. When she feels like wallowing, she reads blogs written by parents whose kids are severely autistic, nonverbal, or have full mutation fragile X syndrome.

She knows she should feel lucky that her boys don't have full mutation fragile X syndrome, but at times she thinks they might as well. "Me and my boys are functioning. But really who would want to be me?"

Mara's family is a classic three-generation fragile X family—three generations of premutation. The grandfather, now with FXTAS, previously with the broad autism phenotype, was withholding, humorless, and disapproving. Mara internalized his disrespect for her, and that, combined with a premutation woman's tendency toward mood and anxiety disorders, led her to dislike herself and, at times, her sons. "I have to accept that they will never be 'normal boys,' but I can't, really." Mara shrinks from conflict, and when she talks about how violent the boys can be, in secret, she seems a bit afraid of them. Meanwhile, the boys, with their high-level premutations, are intellectually intact, but Tommy in particular has many social behaviors common to both full mutation fragile X syndrome and the autism spectrum.

WHAT IT MEANS TO BE NORMAL

Borderlands of diseases shine a light on what it means to be normal and what constitutes disease. A woman with 55 CGG repeats will never be a mother to a child with fragile X syndrome, at least as far as we know now. But a woman with just one more CGG repeat could be. A boy like Matt, who has bipolar disorder, is on five medications to control his mania, but when he takes his medications he is able to go to school and appears to be well. His brother Tommy, in his mother's words, is "obviously strange." But Tommy doesn't have a traditionally recognized disorder. He has the BAP, not autism.

Thinking about the "normal" person and disease got me curious about myself. You can't spend years researching a condition whose symptoms can include everything from anxiety to dementia to nothing and not wonder where you fall on the spectrum of risk.

Randi had been after me for years to get tested for the premutation. As Louise Gane had told me, "She will attribute anything to the premutation." I found it frightening. I thought it quite possible that I was a carrier. I'm an anxious person, and I had autoimmune thyroid disease. My periods had stopped when I was a couple of years short of the US average. As my father aged into his eighties, he developed a tremor, and sometimes fell when he tried to sit down. Maybe he really had FXTAS.

But when I suddenly needed a pacemaker for a slow heart rate, just as my father had, Randi was insistent. Apparently, inclusion bodies related to excess *FMR1* mRNA can affect the sinus node, the part of the heart that sets our heart rate. I needed a pacemaker because my sinus node wasn't functioning normally. "I can't tell you how many people whose brains I've wanted to study who couldn't get into an MRI machine because they had pacemakers," Randi told me. (Pacemakers are often metal and aren't allowed near the MRI machine's giant magnet.)

So I finally decided to get tested. When I went out to Staten Island with Suzanne and Sam to see Sally Nolin, I spent a few minutes in an exam room having my blood drawn. I had to discuss the implications of a positive test with the doctor, particularly the implications for my daughters if I were a premutation carrier. I hadn't thought that through. But there I was with my vein open.

My results took just a few days to come back, because Sally Nolin kindly took a personal interest. I had two *FMR1* alleles, like all women. Both had 29 CGG repeats. Being extra careful, Sally rechecked my sample to make sure she hadn't measured the same allele twice. She hadn't. I was in the sweet spot. Not too many, not too few.

Therefore, just as I would be an obligate premutation carrier if my father had FXTAS, my test proved that my father's tremor and falls were *not* due to FXTAS. If they were, I would have inherited the premutation from him. My sinus node failed because of something called sick sinus syndrome, which only means that something was wrong with my sinus node. My period stopped when I was in my late forties because, well, it just did. And I had thyroid disease because thyroid disease is common, and as a doctor, I know that when you hear hoofbeats, you should think of horses, not zebras. And anxiety? Don't we all have that, at least some of the time?

So none of those problems had anything to do with an *FMR1* mutation, right? But once your eyes have been opened to what a "silent" mutation can do, it keeps you wondering. Maybe my health problems, or even my character, had to do with some as yet unnoticed mutation, another bit of underappreciated DNA.

To me, this relieving result only adds to the mystery of the premutation. How many others are out there, waiting to be discovered?

Until Stephanie Sherman solved her own paradox by showing that the CGG repeat was an unstable string of DNA that did not code for a protein, but could turn off the *FMR1* gene, that string of CGG repeats was considered "nonsense." It seemed to have no purpose. But now we can see that even minor deviations from the normal range—perhaps even the borderlands of the normal range, high or low—can have great consequences.

Chapter Nine

OUTCOMES

THE SOLITARS, the family with the hundred-year saga I introduced in chapter 1, are kind, determined, and generous people who want only the best for their family. They benefited greatly from treatment at the MIND Institute. So why exactly have their lives been so damn hard?

Recall that Mindy and Lowell have three children with full mutation fragile X syndrome, a set of boy twins and a younger girl. Mindy suffers from anxiety, depression, pain, and multiple medical problems. Her relationships with her children, husband, and parents present many challenges. Her mother is disabled as is her grandfather. Her cousin, an alleged gang member, was murdered by his own father.

It's self-evident that even in the absence of additional troubles, having three kids with full mutation fragile X syndrome is the kind of body slam from which you don't just bounce back. But I think there's more to it.

Consider another family I have gotten to know over the years, the Berendts. Laurie and Dan Berendt are also the parents of three children with full mutation fragile X syndrome.[1] The shocking diagnosis was made after the youngest boy, Ian, was born with Down syndrome, which was obvious in the delivery room. Because Laurie had been concerned about the development of her four-year-old son, Mark, the entire family underwent further genetic testing. It revealed that Ian had fragile X syndrome as well as Down syndrome and that Mark and Sarah, his elder sister, had fragile X syndrome.

Ian was severely intellectually disabled and behaviorally disturbed. He was minimally verbal and very hypervigilant, lashing out if anyone came too close, even Laurie. Nonetheless, Laurie and Dan found an accepting community in their church (Ian wore oven mitts to services, so he couldn't scratch and grab) and included Ian in as many aspects of their lives as he could tolerate. When he was a young teen, they made the painful decision to place him into a group home. Both admit that the fact that they agreed on this no-win decision kept their marriage from falling apart.

At the age of twenty-six, Ian died of aspiration pneumonia, an unspeakable loss.

TWO FAMILIES

Though she and Dan grieve, Laurie has remained, essentially, a well premutation carrier. She is athletic and busy and has a rewarding career. "I don't fly the flag of fragile X syndrome too often," she told me, preferring to have an identity outside of being a fragile X mom. She explained that before she had intellectually disabled kids, she was too shy to stand up and introduce her parents in church; but advocating for her kids gave her the confidence she needed for a new career. She now teaches public speaking. She is youthful and attractive and knows how to have fun with her family and with friends—hiking, climbing, mountain biking, and trying craft beers all over her beloved Pacific Northwest. Her son Mark, who is mildly affected by fragile X, adores her and posts lovely pictures of her on Facebook, typically with a pizza on the table in front of her and a mountain range behind.

One of the most remarkable things about Laurie and Dan is the way they accept their children as they are. When Dan, an engineer, told me about the education of his fragile X daughter, Sarah, he said, "College was a *slog*," as though he were describing her completing the Boston Marathon on a cold, rainy day. She had done something that was really hard for her. There was empathy for her struggle and pride in her persistence. The emphasis was on the achievement, despite the difficulty.

Laurie had borne the brunt of Ian's severe behavioral outbursts, and she had tolerated Mark's hyperactivity and her daughter's learning disabilities while providing them the emotional support they needed to grow up with dignity and self-worth. Today, Mark is semi independent and works in a restaurant, while Sarah works with children with special needs.

Just as the Berendts have, Mindy has fought like hell to get appropriate care for her kids, and she adores them just as the Berendts adore theirs. She takes pride in their achievements (both the twins are artists with a great sense of color and space) and values all the children's humor and sass. But in contrast, I observed a lack of cohesion between Mindy and her husband, which may result in an "every man for himself" feeling about this family. Mindy's parents can be a big help, but there is distrust between Mindy and her parents, which goes both ways.

Having said that, the differences between Mindy's experience and Laurie's are not all about family support. In fact, Laurie grew up with her own stresses in the family. Her mother turned against her father when he became ill. Laurie's beloved dad died of complications of FXTAS just after Ian passed away.

These families in fact have many similarities, but the biggest difference between them, as I see it, is the fact that Mindy suffers the effects of the premutation on her *own* body and mind. She has a history of severe anxiety and attention-deficit hyperactivity disorder since childhood. As a teenager, she got sick at parties and was bullied at school. She has type 2 diabetes and Crohn's disease, an autoimmune disorder. She has chronic joint pain related to joint hyperextensibility. She went through early menopause and has early symptoms of FXTAS, including a vocal tremor.

Psychologically, Mindy experiences her life as a constant battle with bureaucracies, reflecting, perhaps, the executive function deficits of the premutation carrier. Without intact executive function, it's very difficult to get things done. As a significantly affected carrier, Mindy has more on her plate than simply being a mother of fragile X kids, as challenging as that is. She has her own multitude of conditions, which make it that much harder to create a positive atmosphere for her family.

In contrast, Laurie makes it look relatively easy. With her executive function intact, her body healthy, and her emotions reasonably stable, she appears to juggle her home, her work, her husband, and her two living children with pleasure.

It's my hypothesis that the differences between families with similar genetic risks have to do with the mind and body of the carrier. Carriers who are more severely affected struggle more when they have fully affected children.

A CONFLUENCE OF INFLUENCES

Donald Bailey, a North Carolina-based psychologist, has linked parental distress and maternal depression to child behavior problems. In other words, he finds that the child's behavior problems cause the mother's depression, and not the other way around.[2] But after years of meeting carriers and their kids, I'm not so sure. This will always be a which-came-first problem. Of course, it's plain common sense that having difficult, even assaultive children in the home would have an adverse impact on the mother who tries to raise them, and more specifically could adversely impact her health. But it is just as reasonable to suppose that the health of the carrier is the most important measure determining quality of life for carriers, spouses, and their children. Someone with significant executive function deficits will have difficulty navigating a stubborn, withholding bureaucracy. A young mother of hyperactive boys who can't stay on her feet because of joint pain will find it hard to maintain an orderly home. A depressed, driven carrier like Margaret (from the previous chapter), whose best psychological defense is a rigid refusal to accept her son's impairment, is not likely to have a good relationship with her fragile X son. Maternal mental health affects the behavior of the entire household.

However, there are other ways, more overtly related to the biology of *FMR1* mutations, to look at the relationship between carrier health and child behavior problems. For example, a carrier within a specific range of CGG repeats could be more prone to mental and physical health problems.

Interestingly, carrier distress—particularly psychological distress and FXPOI—has been linked pretty consistently with having a "midrange" repeat number—60 to 100—as we have seen.[3] A mother with 60 CGG repeats has a slim chance of giving birth to a child with a full mutation. A mother with 80 to 100 repeats, however, has close to a 100 percent chance if her child inherits the mutated X; so in that 80–100 CGG repeat range, there is a high probability of a sensitive, symptomatic mother having at least one full mutation child.

But there are other biological variables that affect carrier well-being besides CGG repeat number. Separately, there is FMRP level. FMRP, or fragile X mental retardation protein, is the necessary ingredient for the developing brain that is absent in boys with full mutation fragile X syndrome, and significantly lowered in girls. In carriers, it varies from person to person, but it tends to decrease as carriers enter the higher range of CGG repeats. As the CGG repeat number increases toward 200 and FMRP decreases, the carrier begins to look more and more like an individual with a full mutation.

For example, Mara's boys, Matt and Tommy, have close to 200 repeats each. They are both highly symptomatic carriers. At least some of their disability is probably related to the lowered FMRP level of the high-level carrier. They are not *intellectually* disabled, but they have some emotional and behavioral features of fragile X syndrome. In particular, Tommy's severe ADHD reflects his poor executive function, and his unusual social behaviors and phobias are more typically present in boys with the full mutation.

Recent work on the subject of high-level premutation carriers has shown that the lowered FMRP level associated with more CGG repeats, combined with the higher *FMR1* mRNA level associated with the premutation, functions as a "double hit," causing both developmental problems and problems associated with neurodegeneration (see chapter 8). Not only does lowered FMRP cause fragile X–like symptoms, but it also affects the amygdala, the "emotional processing area" of the brain. And increased *FMR1* mRNA causes both neurodegenerative problems, such as the tremors and ataxia associated with FXTAS, and is associated with neurodevelopmental problems, such as ADHD and autism spectrum disorders.[4]

Tommy and Matt are boys, and should they father children, their sons will be unaffected, because all sons inherit the Y chromosome from their fathers. But all of Tommy and Matt's daughters will be carriers, and it's likely that they too will have high repeat numbers. Those daughters will also have low FMRP levels. And those daughters may well have children with fragile X syndrome, and they will struggle to raise those intellectually disabled children without a normal level of FMRP themselves.

Then there is the Lyon hypothesis (see chapter 2), which explains how women, despite having two X chromosomes in every single cell, have only one X chromosome that is active in each cell. Female carriers, as a group, have a 50/50 ratio of premutated Xs to normal Xs active in their cells, but in any given individual the ratio can be quite skewed. A carrier could have many more premutated Xs that are active than normal Xs that are active throughout her body. She could be much more affected as a carrier in this way, despite having the same number of CGG repeats as another woman with an opposite ratio.

Another way that factors other than child behavior can influence family outcomes is mate choice. In a concept known as *assortative mating*,[5] it is posited that people tend to choose mates who are like themselves. Having met many premutation carriers and full mutation women, I have found that they tend to marry people with "impairments similar to their own,"[6] as Julia Bell put it. I have never heard of a couple who were *both* premutation carriers, although this does occur, but Mindy and her husband are a good example of a couple with characteristics that are synergistic. Actually, so are Dan and Laurie. Their strengths multiply one another's.

LOOKING BACK: HOW COREY BECAME A VICTIM

Speaking of cause and effect, or to put another spin on it, nature and nurture, let's talk about Corey, Mindy's cousin. His story is the most mysterious in this book. Perhaps the reader is thinking that the biggest mystery is why I would think that the premutation had anything to do with his death. Obviously, he was murdered. What could his premutation have had to do with it?

Almost nothing is known about the genetics of victimization. But much has been written about the *epigenetics* of victimization.[7] Epigenetics, it will be recalled, refers to the impact that life events (nurture) have on when and where genes are expressed (nature). The science of epigenetics has shown us that nature and nurture really can't exist without each other. Life events and genes are always in play, modifying one another.

Take Carol, for example. We saw in chapter 6 how her early years with an abusive father and an ineffectual mother set her up to have emotional difficulties, by direct influence, and at least in theory by epigenetic changes to her gene expression wrought by early childhood deprivation. But Carol has special gifts that not everyone is lucky enough to have. She is brilliant and determined. She compensated for her low self-esteem, as she herself put it, by overachieving.

Corey was not blessed with Carol's capacity to rise above adverse childhood experiences. He is dead, and his mother declined to be interviewed for this book. The information I have about Corey comes from Mindy and Glenn, both of whom spoke freely about his tragic end at the hands of his father. Mindy painted a picture of a young man, diagnosed as a child with Asperger syndrome, whose loneliness and poor sense of self-worth led him to associate with other troubled youths as a means of finding a social life. But he didn't fit into gang culture, either.

He abused substances that included alcohol, methamphetamine, and cocaine. That contributed to his autopsy-confirmed FXTAS and the fact that he already had symptoms of FXTAS, including tremor and gait disturbance, in his thirties.[8]

Thanks to his own involvement in illegal activities, Corey may have been exposed to more disturbing triggers than he would have been otherwise, and more than he was able to process given his condition. According to Dr. Randi Hagerman, people with a premutation who have been exposed to potential sources of trauma may be predisposed to develop PTSD. "They will never forget a trauma," she told me.[9]

People with prior histories of trauma are more likely to experience more trauma. Why might this be? It's complicated, but evidence suggests that the hyperarousal that is characteristic of PTSD can prevent people from responding to new stressors effectively.[10] Thus, the more someone is victimized, the less likely he is to have an appropriate response to a new threat. His capacity to respond to threats, so to speak, has already been maxed out. Emotional numbing and an expectation that one's life will be shortened—perhaps in Corey's case, a self-fulfilling prophecy—are criteria that psychiatrists use to diagnose PTSD.

Still, what does Corey's premutation have to do with his being shot to death?

A person who suffers from poor executive function is a setup to be a victim. People with executive function deficits don't think and plan in an organized, linear way. They have difficulty incorporating and responding to new information. Like Mindy in her dream, when she danced on the *Titanic* as she drowned, the premutation carrier with severe executive dysfunction can feel helpless, trapped by fate. Inflexible, she has already lost the struggle.

Then, let's be honest, Corey was not an innocent bystander when he died. His father, Leo, told the authorities that while they were preparing dinner at a campsite in Michigan, he went to get a steak to put on the fire, and that when he left, all was well. When he returned, Corey attacked him, unprovoked. We will never know what Corey was thinking—or for that matter, whether what Corey's father told the court was even true. But a recent case series of fourteen people with a mixed premutation/full mutation picture showed a high incidence of mood disorders and impulse control disorders.[11] Corey's was one of the cases discussed. He had been diagnosed with bipolar disorder, substance abuse, and acute stress disorder. As a child, he was said to have learning disabilities, impulsivity, and labile (rapidly shifting) mood. All of these combined could have been a recipe for a rageful outburst.

Again, we don't know exactly what happened. But we do know that there was a confrontation, and Leo was carrying a gun.

To be sure, the huge majority of murder victims are not premutation carriers, and the huge majority of premutation carriers are never murdered. But somewhere between nature and nurture, the premutation was the theme of Corey's life story—and it was there at his end.

WHAT CAN CARRIERS DO?

The answer is not "nothing." Although there is no specific treatment for FXTAS (see chapter 5) and there is no cure for FXPOI (see chapter 4), much can be done to ameliorate symptoms, even to the point of restoring fertility in FXPOI. The neuropsychiatric symptoms of FXAND, such as depression and anxiety, are quite treatable with medications and different psychotherapies. A 2014 review by Jonathan Polussa, Andrea Schneider, and Randi Hagerman rounds up the steps a premutation carrier can take to protect his or her health and minimize premutation-related illness.[12]

The authors begin with ideas for stimulating neurogenesis, meaning the growth of new nerve cells in the brain. SSRI antidepressants have been shown to do this, and even simpler, so has exercise.

Next, and slightly more complicated to understand, is the idea of reducing oxidative stress. In the brain and elsewhere, oxidation reactions take place in the mitochondria, tiny organelles that provide the cell with energy to function. Unfortunately, oxidation reactions produce the colorfully named "free radicals," which can be damaging to the cell. When these free radicals overwhelm the cell's protective antioxidants, the cell is under oxidative stress. Oxidative stress is known to be a factor in neurodegenerative diseases like Parkinson's and Alzheimer's and in many inflammatory conditions.

Treatment for oxidative stress consists of neutralizing free radicals by replenishing the body's diminished supply of antioxidants; in other words, it's a healthy diet rich in vitamins, minerals, fruits and vegetables, and foods especially high in antioxidants, like green tea. Several drugs that protect the mitochondria are also in development.

The authors further advise the carrier to treat conditions that contribute to brain aging in all of us. For example, premutation carriers should quit smoking, limit alcohol and drug use, and avoid exposure to toxins. Obesity, high blood pressure, and sleep apnea should be assessed and treated. It's important to treat depression, anxiety, and pain—not just because these are bad for your brain, but also to improve quality of life. Finally, meditation and biofeedback can decrease stress, and cognitive training can keep the brain young. All of these are low-tech, already

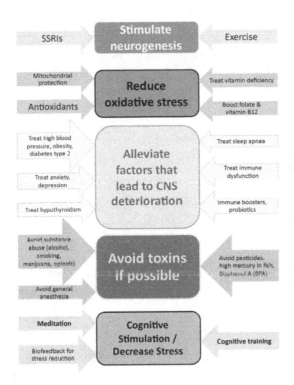

FIGURE 9.1 Recommendations to support healthy aging for *FMR1* premutation carriers.

Jonathan Polussa, Andrea Schneider, and Randi Hagerman, "Molecular Advances Leading to Treatment Implications for Fragile X Premutation Carriers," *Brain Disorders and Therapy* 3 (2014): 1000119.

invented treatments that address brain dysfunction, and they can be adopted by anyone so motivated.

A MUTATION'S TRANSFORMATION

Early on in my research, I interviewed historian and sociologist Daniel Navon, who studies the history of genetic disease. He pointed out the transformation of the *meaning* of the fragile X premutation: how it has morphed, conceptually, from a mere "carrier" gene with no consequences for the carrier to a gene that confers a high risk of two rare adult-onset disorders— FXTAS and FXPOI—and has more recently been found to contribute to a group of relatively common conditions (the broad autism phenotype for one, and psychiatric disorders such as anxiety) that may manifest from infancy on, in those affected. It is likely that over the next several years, as research continues and genetic testing is increasingly available, more and more people will be found to be affected by these and other previously unnoticed new problems. In other words, carriers will become "patients."

Navon told me, "None of this would have been recognized if it weren't for the incredible work the fragile X syndrome community has done to bring patients, their families, clinicians and researchers together."[13] I could not agree more. The story of the premutation and its transition from invisible carrier state to significant condition is written by the individuals who discovered it and the individuals who have suffered—or not—from its effects on their minds and bodies.

Every person profiled in *The Carriers* has his or her own narrative. Nonetheless, I have endeavored to show that the narratives of the doctors, scientists, families, and patients in this book are inseparable. In the complex world of genetics and behavior, only the summation of innumerable biographies can produce meaningful hypotheses. Every life story brings you closer to the truth.

NOTES

INTRODUCTION

1. Patel is a pseudonym. Some details have been changed for anonymity and clarity.
2. Jessie is also a pseudonym. Her personal details and her father's have been changed for anonymity and clarity.
3. David Hessl, interview, September 30, 2015.

1. ONE DAMN THING AFTER ANOTHER

1. This chapter is based on interviews conducted with the Solitar family over a three-day period in May 2018. All patients' names are pseudonyms, and some minor identifying details have been changed for anonymity and clarity. Additional information was obtained from a self-published book by Mindy and Lowell Solitar, *Surviving Fragile X*, and from reviews of the Solitar family's medical charts, with their permission.
2. Randi J. Hagerman, personal communication, May 5, 2021.
3. Molly Losh, "Social Cognition," lecture, 2nd Annual Conference on *FMR1* Premutation, Sitges, Spain, October 1, 2015.
4. Anne C. Wheeler, John Sideris, Randi Hagerman, Elizabeth Berry-Kravis, Flora Tassone, and Donald B. Bailey Jr., "Developmental Profiles

of Infants with an *FMR1* Premutation," *Journal of Neurodevelopmental Disorders* 8 (2016): 40.

5. James Bourgeois, interview, September 2015.

6. Temple Grandin, *Thinking in Pictures: And Other Reports From My Life With Autism* (New York: Doubleday, 1995).

7. Randi J. Hagerman, Maureen Leehey, W. Heinrichs, Flora Tassone, R. Wilson, J. Hills, Jim Grigsby, B. Gage, and Paul J. Hagerman, "Intention Tremor, Parkinsonism, and Generalized Brain Atrophy in Male Carriers of Fragile X," *Neurology* 57 (2001): 127–30.

8. Paul Hagerman, lecture, September 30, 2015.

9. Randi J. Hagerman, Dragana Protic, Akash Rajaratnam, Maria J. Salcedo-Arellano, Elber Yuksel Aydin, and Andrea Schneider, "Fragile X–Associated Neuropsychiatric Disorders (FXAND)," *Frontiers in Psychiatry* 9 (2018): 564.

10. Verónica Martínez-Cerdeño, Mirna Lechpammer, Aisha Lott, Andrea Schneider, and Randi Hagerman, "Fragile X–Associated Tremor/Ataxia Syndrome in a Man in His 30s," *Journal of the American Medical Association: Neurology* 72, no. 9 (September 1, 2015): 1070–73.

11. Information on file.

2. FRAGILE X MUTATIONS

1. Giovanni Neri, "The Clinical Phenotype of the Fragile X Syndrome and Related Disorders," in *Fragile X Syndrome: From Genetics to Targeted Treatment*, ed. Rob Willemson and R. Frank Kooy (San Diego, CA: Academic Press, 2017), 3–18.

2. Denise Cook, Scott A. Cameron, and Emma V. Jones, "Fragile X Mental Retardation Protein: Regulator of Specific mRNAs or Master Regulator of Global Translation," *Journal of Neuroscience* 30, no. 21 (2010): 7121–23.

3. Randi J. Hagerman, interview, October 1, 2015.

4. Peter S. Harper, *A Short History of Medical Genetics* (New York: Oxford University Press, 2008).

5. Harper, *Short History of Medical Genetics*.

6. Marsha L. Richmond, "The 'Domestication' of Heredity: The Familial Organization of Geneticists at Cambridge University, 1895–1910," *Journal of the History of Biology* 39, no. 3 (2006): 574.

7. Marsha L. Richmond, "Women as Mendelians and Geneticists," *Science & Education* 24, nos. 1–2 (2015): 125–50.

8. Richmond, "Women as Mendelians," 135.
9. James D. Watson, *The Double Helix: A Personal Account of the Discovery of the Structure of DNA* (London: Weidenfeld & Nicolson, 1981).
10. Harper, *Short History of Medical Genetics*.
11. Mary F. Lyon, "Gene Action in the X-Chromosome of the Mouse (Mus musculus L.)," *Nature* 190 (1961): 372–73.
12. Sarah Bundey, "Julia Bell MRCS LRCP FRCP (1879–1979): Steamboat Lady, Statistician and Geneticist," *Journal of Medical Biography* 4 (1996): 8–13.
13. Bundey, "Julia Bell," 10.
14. Reed E. Pyeritz, "The Family History: The First Genetic Test, and Still Useful After All These Years?" *Journal of Genetic Medicine* 14, no. 1 (2012): 3–9, 4.
15. Bundey, "Julia Bell," 11.
16. *Journal of the American Medical Association* 58, no. 25 (1912): 1966.
17. Julia Bell, "Plural Births with a New Pedigree," *Biometrika* 25, nos. 1–2 (1933): 110–20, 119.
18. J. Purdon Martin and Julia Bell, "A Pedigree of Mental Deficiency Showing Sex-Linkage," *Journal of Neurological Psychiatry* 6, nos. 3–4 (1943): 154–57.
19. Siddhartha Mukherjee, *The Gene* (New York: Simon & Schuster, 2016).
20. Randi J. Hagerman, Elizabeth Berry-Kravis, Heather Cody Hazlett, Donald B. Bailey Jr., Herve Moine, R. Frank Kooy, Flora Tassone, et al., "Fragile X Syndrome," *Nature Reviews Disease Primers* 3 (2017): 17065.
21. David L. Nelson, Michael R. Santoro, and Stephen T. Warren, "Fragile X Syndrome Genetics," in Willemson and Kooy, *Fragile X Syndrome*, 19–39.
22. David S. Moore, *The Developing Genome* (New York: Oxford University Press, 2015), 40–41.
23. Gillian Turner, "Historical Overview of X-Linked Mental Retardation," in *The Fragile X Syndrome: Diagnosis, Biochemistry and Intervention*, ed. Randi J. Hagerman and Pam McKenzie (Denver: Spectra, 1983), 1–16.
24. Robert Gordon Lehrke, "X-Linked Mental Retardation and Verbal Disability," in *Birth Defects: Original Article Series* (New York: National Foundation, March of Dimes, 1974), 1.
25. William Bateson MS Add.8634/B.27: Letter to the Zoologist Adam Sedgwick Coining the Term "Genetics," 1905. Cambridge Digital Archive, https://cudl.lib.cam.ac.uk/collections/batesonarchive/1 (accessed August 5, 2021).

26. Lehrke, "X-Linked Mental Retardation."

27. Turner, "Historical Overview."

28. Andrea Prader, "Testicular Size: Assessment and Clinical Importance," *Triangle: The Sandoz Journal of Medical Science* 7, no. 6 (1966): 240–43.

29. Turner, "Historical Overview."

30. Turner, "Historical Overview," 12.

31. Lehrke, "X-Linked Mental Retardation," 10–11.

32. Lehrke, "X-Linked Mental Retardation," 72.

33. Lehrke, "X-Linked Mental Retardation," 72.

34. Lehrke, "X-Linked Mental Retardation," 77.

35. Lehrke, "X-Linked Mental Retardation," 80.

36. Roger E. Stevenson and Charles E. Schwartz, "X-Linked Intellectual Disability: Unique Vulnerability of the Male Genome," *Developmental Disabilities Research Reviews* 15, no. 4 (2009): 361–68.

37. B.W. Richards, P.E. Sylvester, and C. Brooker, "Fragile X-Linked Mental Retardation: The Martin-Bell Syndrome," *Journal of Mental Deficiencies Research* 25 (1981): 253–56.

38. John Opitz, "On the Gates of Hell and a Most Unusual Gene," *American Journal of Medical Genetics* 23 (1986): 1–10.

39. Giovanni Neri and John M. Opitz, "Sixty Years of X-Linked Mental Retardation: A Historical Footnote," *American Journal of Medical Genetics* 97, no. 3 (2000): 231.

3. VILLAGE OF FOOLS

1. Sergio Villada, interview, October 24, 2016.

2. Villada interview.

3. Gustavo Alvarez Gardeazabal, *El divino* (Bogotá: Plaza & Janes, 1986).

4. Wilmar Saldarriaga Gil, Randi J. Hagerman, María Jimena Salcedo, Flora Tassone, Julián Ramirez-Cheyne, and Marisol Silva, "Fragile X Syndrome in a Colombian Family," *Iatreia* 31, no. 1 (2018): 76–85.

5. Wilmar Saldarriaga Gil, interview, November 16, 2016.

6. Wilmar Saldarriaga Gil, José Vicente Forero Forero, Laura Yuriko González Teshima, Carlos A. Fandiño Losada, and Carolina Isaza, "Ricaurte," in *Fragile X Syndrome in Ricaurte, Colombia*, ed. Wilmar Saldarriaga Gil (Cali, Colombia: Universidad del Valle Programa Editorial, 2018), 55.

7. José Vicente Forero Forero, Laura Yuriko González Teshima, and Wilmar Saldarriaga Gil, "Genealogies in the Families with Fragile X Syndrome in Ricaurte,"in Saldarriaga Gil, *Fragile X Syndrome in Ricaurte*, 104–5.

8. Forero Forero, González Teshima, and Saldarriaga Gil, "Genealogies in the Families with Fragile X Syndrome in Ricaurte," 111.

9. Saldarriaga Gil et al., "Ricaurte," 58.

10. Wilmar Saldarriaga Gil, interview, February 18, 2020.

11. All patients' names are pseudonyms. Minor details have been changed for anonymity and clarity.

12. Wilmar Saldarriaga, Pamela Lein, Laura Yuriko González Teshima, Carolina Isaza, Lina Rosa, Andrew Polyak, Randi Hagerman, et al., "Phenobarbital Use and Neurological Problems in *FMR1* Premutation Carriers," *Neurotoxicology* 53 (2016): 141–47.

13. Wilmar Saldarriaga Gil, interview, February 17, 2020.

14. Sarah L. Nolin, Anne Glicksman, Nicole Tortora, Emily Allen, James Macpherson, Montserrat Mila, Angela M. Vianna-Morgante, et al., "Expansions and Contractions of the FMR1 CGG Repeat in 5,508 Transmissions of Normal, Intermediate, and Premutation Alleles," *American Journal of Medical Genetics* 179A (2019): 1148–56.

15. Ying-Hui Fu, Derek P.A. Kuhl, Antonio Pizzuti, Maura Pieretti, James S. Sutcliffe, Stephen Richards, Annemieke J.M.H.Verkerk, et al., "Variation of the CGG Repeat at the Fragile X Site Results in Genetic Instability: Resolution of the Sherman Paradox," *Cell* 67 (1991): 1047–58.

16. Villada interview.

17. Bruce G. Charlton, "Crick's Gossip Test and Watson's Boredom Principle: A Pseudo-Mathematical Analysis of Effort in Scientific Research," *Medical Hypotheses* 70, no. 1 (2008): 1–3.

4. A CLASSIC ZEBRA

1. Ariel and the names of her family members are pseudonyms. Some minor details have been changed for anonymity and clarity.

2. Belle, interview, December 14, 2017.

3. Carly Heyman, *My eXtra Special Brother* (Marietta: Fragile X Association of GA, 2003).

4. Stephanie Sherman, interview, December 18, 2017.

5. Amy Cronister, interview, January 22, 2018.
6. A. Cronister, R. Schreiner, M. Wittenberger, K. Amiri, K. Harris, and R.J. Hagerman, "Heterozygous Fragile X Female: Historical, Physical, Cognitive, and Cytogenetic Features," *American Journal of Medical Genetics* 38 (1991): 269–74.
7. Stephanie Sherman, interview, December 18, 2017.
8. Stephanie L. Sherman, "Premature Ovarian Failure in the Fragile X Syndrome," *American Journal of Medical Genetics* 97 (2000): 189–94.
9. Lawrence M. Nelson, "Primary Ovarian Insufficiency," *New England Journal of Medicine* 360, no. 6 (February 5, 2009): 606–14.
10. E. Allen, A.K. Sullivan, M. Marcus, C. Small, C. Dominguez, M.P. Epstein, K. Charen, et al., "Examination of Reproductive Aging Milestones Among Women Who Carry the FMR1 Premutation," *Human Reproduction* 22, no. 8 (August 2007): 2142–52.
11. American College of Obstetricians and Gynecologists, Committee Opinion, "Hormone Therapy in Primary Ovarian Insufficiency," no. 698, May 2017.
12. J. Ryan, J. Scali, Isabelle Carriere, H. Amieva, O. Rouaud, C. Berr, K. Ritchie, and M-L. Ancelin, "Impact of a Premature Menopause on Cognitive Function in Later Life," *British Journal of Gynecology* 121, no. 13 (December 2014): 1729–39.
13. Tri Indah Winarni, Weerasak Chonchaiya, Tanjung Ayu Sumekar, Paul Ashwood, Guadalupe Mendoza Morales, Flora Tassone, Danh V. Nguyen, et al., "Immune-Mediated Disorders Among Women Carriers of Fragile X Premutation Alleles," *American Journal of Medical Genetics Part A* 158A (2012): 2473–81.
14. Sonya Campbell, Sarah E.A. Eley, Andrew G. McKechanie, and Andrew C. Stanfield, "Endocrine Dysfunction in Female FMR1 Premutation Carriers: Characteristics and Association with Ill Health," *Genes (Basel)* 7, no. 11 (November 2016).
15. Nelson, "Primary Ovarian Insufficiency."
16. Lawrence M. Nelson, interview, November 20, 2019.
17. Robert H. Brook, "A Physician = Emotion + Passion + Science," *Journal of the American Medical Association* 304, no. 22 (December 8, 2010): 2528–29.
18. C.M. Joachim, C.M. Eads, L. Persani, P. Yurttas Beim, and L.M. Nelson, "An Open Letter to the Primary Ovarian Insufficiency Community," *Minerva Obstetrics and Gynecology* 66, no. 5 (Oct 2014): 519–20.

19. Daisy (pseudonym), email to author, January 8, 2020.

20. Mary Davis, June L. Ventura, Mary Wieners, Sharon N. Covington, Vien H. Vanderhoof, Mary E. Ryan, Deloris E. Koziol, et al., "The Psychosocial Transition Associated with Spontaneous 46,XX Primary Ovarian Insufficiency: Illness Uncertainty, Stigma, Goal Flexibility, and Purpose in Life as Factors in Emotional Health," *Fertility and Sterility* 93, no. 7 (May 1, 2010): 2321–29.

21. Lawrence M. Nelson, "One World, One Woman: A Transformational Leader's Approach to Primary Ovarian Insufficiency," *Menopause* 18, no. 5 (May 2011): 480–87.

22. D. Singer, E. Mann, M.S. Hunter, J. Pitkin, and N. Panay, "The Silent Grief: Psychosocial Aspects of Premature Ovarian Failure," *Climacteric* 1, no. 4 (2011): 428–37.

23. Peter J. Schmidt, Jamie A. Luff, Nazli A. Haq, Vien H. Vanderhoof, Deloris E. Koziol, Karim A. Calis, David R. Rubinow, and Lawrence M. Nelson, "Depression in Women with Spontaneous 46, XX Primary Ovarian Insufficiency," *Journal of Clinical Endocrinology & Metabolism* 96, no. 2 (February 2011): E278–87.

24. Shweta A. Bhatt, "Prolonged Time to Diagnosis of Primary Ovarian Insufficiency (POI) in an Urban Reproductive Endocrinology (RE) Clinic," *Fertility and Sterility* 112, no. 3 (September 2019) Supplement: e354.

25. Etienne Wenger, *Communities of Practice: Learning, Meaning, and Identity* (Cambridge: Cambridge University Press, 1998).

26. Daisy, email to author, January 8, 2020.

27. Ariel, interview, October 25, 2019.

28. Ariel, email to author, November 2, 2019.

29. American College of Obstetricians and Gynecologists, "Hormone Therapy in Primary Ovarian Insufficiency," no. 698, May 2017.

30. Emily C. Corrigan, Margarita J. Raygada, Vien H. Vanderhoof, and Lawrence M. Nelson, "A Woman with Spontaneous Premature Ovarian Failure Gives Birth to a Child with Fragile X Syndrome," *Fertility and Sterility* 84, no. 5 (November 2005): 1508.e5–e8.

31. Karen Usdin, Renate K. Hukema, and Stephanie L. Sherman, "Model Systems for Understanding FXPOI," in *FXTAS, FXPOI, and Other Premutation Disorders*, ed. F. Tassone and D. Hall (Cham, Switzerland: Springer International, 2016), 225–40.

32. Jessica Ezzell Hunter, Michael P. Epstein, Stuart W. Tinker, Krista H. Charen, and Stephanie L. Sherman, "Fragile X–Associated Primary Ovarian Insufficiency: Evidence for Additional Genetic Contributions to Severity," *Genetic Epidemiology* 32, no. 6 (September 2008): 553–59.

33. Allen et al., "Examination of Reproductive Aging Milestones."

34. John J. DeCaro, Celia Dominguez, and Stephanie L. Sherman, "Reproductive Health of Adolescent Girls Who Carry the FMR1 Premutation: Expected Phenotype Based on Current Knowledge of Fragile X–Associated Primary Ovarian Insufficiency," *Annals of the New York Academy of Sciences* 1135 (2008): 99–111.

35. Nelson, "Primary Ovarian Insufficiency."

36. Heather S. Hipp, Krista H. Charen, Jessica B. Spencer, Emily G. Allen, and Stephanie L. Sherman, "Reproductive and Gynecologic Care of Women with Fragile X Primary Ovarian Insufficiency (FXPOI)," *Menopause* 23, no. 9 (September 2016): 993–99.

37. Hilary Hipp, interview, December 2, 2019.

38. Amy Talboy, interview, December 3, 2019.

39. Hipp et al., "Reproductive and Gynecologic Care," 997.

40. Dorothy A. Fink, Lawrence M. Nelson, Reed Pyeritz, Josh Johnson, Stephanie L. Sherman, Yoram Cohen, and Shai E. Elizur, "Fragile X Associated Primary Ovarian Insufficiency (FXPOI): Case Report and Literature Review," *Frontiers in Genetics* 9 (November 2018): 529.

41. Nelson, "One World, One Woman."

42. Franklin, interview, November 16, 2019.

43. James Surowiecki, *The Wisdom of Crowds: Why the Many Are Smarter Than the Few and How Collective Wisdom Shapes Business, Economies, Societies and Nations* (New York: Doubleday, 2004).

44. Surowiecki, *The Wisdom of Crowds*, 167.

45. Surowiecki, *The Wisdom of Crowds*, 160.

46. Franklin interview.

5. THE MOVEMENT DISORDER THAT
STARTED A MOVEMENT

1. Keller is a pseudonym. Some details of all family members have been changed for anonymity and clarity. Later in the chapter, Clay, Jennifer, Cal, and Vivian are also pseudonyms, and again some details have been changed.

2. Sébastien Jacquemont, Randi J. Hagerman, Maureen A. Leehey, Deborah A. Hall, Richard A. Levine, James A. Brunberg, Lin Zhang, et al., "Penetrance of the Fragile X–Associated Tremor/Ataxia Syndrome in a Premutation Carrier Population," *Journal of the American Medical Association* 291, no. 4 (January 28, 2004): 460–69.

3. Annie, interview, August 2, 2016.

4. I have conducted numerous interviews with Dr. Randi J. Hagerman over the phone and in person on many different occasions between May 2015 and September 2020.

5. Randi J. Hagerman and Paul J. Hagerman, lecture, University of California at Davis Medical Center, November 17, 2016.

6. Louise Gane, interview, November 27, 2017.

7. Gane interview.

8. Randi J. Hagerman, interview, November 13, 2017.

9. Hagerman interview.

10. Paul J. Hagerman, lecture, University of California at Davis Medical Center, November 17, 2016.

11. Jennifer, interview, December 3, 2017.

12. Flora Tassone, interview, November 7, 2017.

13. Randi J. Hagerman, Maureen Leehey, W. Heinrichs, Flora Tassone, R. Wilson, J. Hills, J. Grigsby, B. Gage, and Paul J. Hagerman, "Intention Tremor, Parkinsonism, and Generalized Brain Atrophy in Male Carriers of Fragile X," *Neurology* 57, no. 1 (2001): 127–30.

14. Flora Tassone, Randi J. Hagerman, Annette K. Taylor, Louise W. Gane, Tony E. Godfrey, and Paul J. Hagerman, "Elevated Levels of FMR1 mRNA in Carrier Males: A New Mechanism of Involvement in the Fragile-X Syndrome," *American Journal of Human Genetics* 66, no. 1 (January 2000): 6–15.

15. Paul J. Hagerman, interview, September 30, 2015.

16. C.M. Greco, Randi J. Hagerman, Flora Tassone, A.E. Chudley, M.R. Del Bigio, Sébastien Jacquemont, Maureen Leehey, and Paul J. Hagerman, "Neuronal Intranuclear Inclusions in a New Cerebellar Tremor/Ataxia Syndrome Among Fragile X Carriers," *Brain* 125, no. 8 (August 2002): 1760–71.

17. Peter K. Todd, Seok Yoon Oh, Amy Krans, Fang He, Chantal Sellier, Michelle Frazer, Abigail J. Renoux, Kai-chun Chen, et al., "CGG Repeat-Associated Translation Mediates Neurodegeneration in Fragile X Tremor Ataxia Syndrome," *Neuron* 78 (2013): 440–55.

18. Chantal Sellier, Ronald A.M. Buijsen, Fang He, Sam Natla, Laura Jung, Philippe Tropel, Angeline Gaucherot, et al., "Translation of Expanded CGG Repeats into FMRpolyG Is Pathogenic and May Contribute to Fragile X Tremor Ataxia Syndrome," *Neuron* 93, no. 2 (January 18, 2017): 331–47.

19. Peter Todd, interview, September 26, 2019.

20. Vivian, interview, December 13, 2017.

21. Jim Grigsby, Andreea L. Seritan, James A. Bourgeois, Anson Kairys, "FXTAS: Neuropsychological and Neuropsychiatric Phenotypes," in *FXTAS, FXPOI, and Other Premutation Disorders*, ed. Flora Tassone and Deborah Hall (Cham, Switzerland: Springer International, 2016), 42.

22. Elkhonon Goldberg, ed., *Executive Functions in Health and Disease* (San Diego, CA: Academic Press, 2017).

23. Angela G. Brega, Glenn Goodrich, Rachael E. Bennett, David Hessl, Karen Engle, Maureen A. Leehey, Lanee S. Bounds, et al., "The Primary Cognitive Deficit Among Males with Fragile X–Associated Tremor/Ataxia Syndrome (FXTAS) Is a Dysexecutive Syndrome," *Journal of Clinical Experimental Neuropsychology* 30, no. 8 (November 2008): 853–69.

24. Daniel S. Weisholtz, John F. Sullivan, Aaron P. Nelson, Kirk R. Daffner, and David A. Silbersweig, "Cognitive, Emotional, and Behavioral Flexibility and Perseveration in Neuropsychiatric Illness," in Goldberg, *Executive Functions*, 220.

25. Khaled Amiri, Randi J. Hagerman, and Paul A. Hagerman, "Fragile X–Associated Tremor/Ataxia Syndrome: An Aging Face of the Fragile X Gene," *Archives of Neurology* 65, no. 1 (2008): 19–25.

26. Deborah A. Hall, Rachael C. Birch, Mathieu Anheim, Aia E. Jønch, Elizabeth Pintado, Joanne O'Keefe, Julian N. Trollor, et al., "Emerging Topics in FXTAS," *Journal of Neurodevelopmental Disorders* 6 (2014): 31.

27. Steve Warren, interview, January 3, 2018.

28. Peng Jin, interview, December 2, 2019.

29. Randi J. Hagerman and Paul Hagerman, "Fragile X–Associated Tremor/Ataxia Syndrome—Features, Mechanisms, and Management," *Nature Reviews Neurology* 12 (July 2016): 403–12.

30. Ana María Cabal-Herrera, Nattaporn Tassanakijpanich, María Jimena Salcedo-Arellano, and Randi J. Hagerman, "Fragile X–Associated Tremor/

Ataxia Syndrome (FXTAS): Pathophysiology and Clinical Implications," *International Journal of Molecular Sciences* 21 (2020): 4391.
31. Louise Gane, interview, January 8, 2018.

6. ONCE MORE, WITH FEELINGS

1. Randi J. Hagerman, Dragana Protic, Akash Rajaratnam, María J. Salcedo-Arellano, Elber Yuksel Aydin, and Andrea Schneider, "Fragile X–Associated Neuropsychiatric Disorders (FXAND)," *Frontiers in Psychiatry* 9 (2018): 564.
2. Steve Warren, interview, January 3, 2018.
3. David A. Grimes and Kenneth F. Schultz, "Bias and Causal Associations in Observational Research," *Lancet* 359 (2002): 248–52.
4. Stephanie Sherman, interview, December 18, 2017.
5. Randi J. Hagerman, interview, July 1, 2016.
6. Carol is a pseudonym, as are the names of the other members of Carol's family. Minor details have been changed for anonymity and clarity. Interviews with Carol took place over the course of several years by phone and in person on January 19–20, 2020.
7. Amy, interview, November 15, 2016.
8. Verónica Martínez-Cerdeño, Mirna Lechpammer, Aisha Lott, Andrea Schneider, and Randi Hagerman, "Fragile X–Associated Tremor/Ataxia Syndrome in a Man in His 30s," *Journal of the American Medical Association: Neurology* 72, no. 9 (September 1, 2015): 1070–73.
9. Jim Grigsby, Kim Cornish, Darren Hocking, Claudine Kraan, John M. Olichney, Susan M. Rivera, Andrea Schneider, et al., "The Cognitive Neuropsychological Phenotype of Carriers of the *FMR1* Premutation," *Journal of Neurodevelopmental Disorders* 6 (2014): 28.
10. Anne C. Wheeler, Donald B. Bailey Jr., Elizabeth Berry-Kravis, Jan Greenberg, Molly Losh, Marsha Mailick, Montserrat Milà, et al., "Associated Features in Females with an *FMR1* Premutation," *Journal of Neurodevelopmental Disorders* 6 (2014): 30.
11. Audra M. Sterling, Marsha Mailick, Jan Greenberg, Steven F. Warren, and Nancy Brady, "Language Dysfluencies in Females with the *FMR1* Premutation," *Brain and Cognition* 82, no. 1 (2013): 84–89.
12. Cary S. Kogan, Jeremy Turk, Randi J. Hagerman, and Kim M. Cornish, "Impact of the Fragile X Mental Retardation 1 (*FMR1*) Gene Premutation

on Neuropsychiatric Functioning in Adult Males Without Fragile X–Associated Tremor/Ataxia Syndrome: A Controlled Study," *American Journal of Medical Genetics B: Neuropsychiatric Genetics* 147B, no. 6 (September 5, 2008): 859–72.

13. Marsha Mailick Seltzer, Erin T. Barker, Jan S. Greenberg, Jinkuk Hong, Christopher Coe, and David Almeida, "Differential Sensitivity to Life Stress in *FMR1* Premutation Carrier Mothers of Children with Fragile X Syndrome," *Health Psychology* 31, no. 5 (September 2012): 612–22.

14. James A. Bourgeois, Sarah M. Coffey, Susan M. Rivera, David Hessl, Louise W. Gane, Flora Tassone, Claudia Greco, et al., "A Review of Fragile X Premutation Disorders: Expanding the Psychiatric Perspective," *Journal of Clinical Psychiatry* 70, no. 6 (June 2009): 852–62.

15. Arezoo Movaghar, David Page, Murray Brilliant, Mei Wang Baker, Jan Greenberg, Jinkuk Hong, Leann Smith DaWalt, et al., "Data-Driven Phenotype Discovery of *FMR1* Premutation Carriers in a Population-Based Sample," *Science Advances* 5, no. 8 (August 21, 2019): eaaw7195.

16. Marsha Mailick, interview, February 5, 2020.

17. https://www.fragilex.eu/fxpac-2/, February 1, 2020.

18. Donald W. Winnicott, *Playing and Reality* (New York: Penguin, 1971).

19. David S. Moore, *The Developing Genome* (New York: Oxford University Press, 2015).

20. Moore, *The Developing Genome*, 185.

21. Rob Willemson and R. Frank Kooy, eds., *Fragile X Syndrome: From Genetics to Targeted Treatment* (Cham, Switzerland: Elsevier, 2017), 5.

22. Moore, *The Developing Genome*, 14.

23. M.J. Meaney, D.H. Aitken, C. van Berkel, S. Bhatnagar, and R.M. Sapolsky, "Effect of Neonatal Handling on Age-Related Impairments Associated with the Hippocampus," *Science* 239, no. 4841, Pt. 1 (February 12, 1988): 766–68.

24. K. Braun and F.A. Champagne, "Paternal Influences on Offspring Development: Behavioural and Epigenetic Pathways," *Journal of Neuroendocrinology* 26, no. 10 (October 2014): 697–706.

25. E.R. deKloet, "Brain Corticosteroid Receptor Balance and Homeostatic Control," *Frontiers in Neuroendocrinology* 12 (1991): 95–164.

26. Julia I. Herzog and Christian Schmahl, "Adverse Childhood Experiences and the Consequences on Neurobiological, Psychosocial, and Somatic Conditions Across the Lifespan," *Frontiers in Psychiatry* 9 (2018): 420.

27. Mingyi Chen and Rebecca E. Lacey, "Adverse Childhood Experiences and Adult Inflammation: Findings from the 1958 British Birth Cohort," *Brain, Behavior, and Immunity* 69 (March 2018): 582–90.

28. Natalie J. Sachs-Ericsson, Julia L. Sheffler, Ian H. Stanley, Jennifer R. Piazza, and Kristopher J. Preacher, "When Emotional Pain Becomes Physical: Adverse Childhood Experiences, Pain, and the Role of Mood and Anxiety Disorders," *Journal of Clinical Psychology* 73, no. 10 (October 2017): 1403–28.

29. Gretchen E. Tietjen, Jan L. Brandes, B. Lee Peterlin, Arnolda Eloff, Rima M. Dafer, Michael R. Stein, Ellen Drexler, et al., "Childhood Maltreatment and Migraine (Part I): Prevalence and Adult Revictimization—A Multicenter Headache Clinic Survey," *Headache* 50, no. 1 (January 2010): 20–31.

30. Ann Polcari, Keren Rabi, Elizabeth Bolger, and Martin H. Teicher, "Parental Verbal Affection and Verbal Aggression in Childhood Differentially Influence Psychiatric Symptoms and Wellbeing in Young Adulthood," *Child Abuse and Neglect* 38, no. 1 (January 2014): 91–102.

31. Jeewook Choi, "Preliminary Evidence for White Matter Tract Abnormalities in Young Adults Exposed to Parental Verbal Abuse," *Biological Psychiatry* 65, no. 3 (February 1, 2009): 227–34.

32. Julie L. Crouch, Erin R. McKay, Gabriela Lelakowska, Regina Hiraoka, Ericka Rutledge, David J. Bridgett, and Joel S. Milner, "Do Emotion Regulation Difficulties Explain the Association Between Executive Functions and Child Physical Abuse Risk?" *Child Abuse and Neglect* 80 (June 2018): 99–107.

33. Amy, interview, November 15, 2016.

34. Louise Ganc, interview, January 8, 2018.

7. WHAT ARE FRAGILE EGGS?

1. Suzanne is a pseudonym, as are the names of her family members. Minor details have been changed for anonymity and clarity.

2. Suzanne, interview, 2015.

3. Sarah Nolin, interview, June 8, 2017.

4. Isabel Fernandez-Carvajal, Blanca Lopez Posadas, Ruiqin Pan, Christopher Raske, Paul J. Hagerman, and Flora Tassone, "Expansion of an FMR1 Grey-Zone Allele to a Full Mutation in Two Generations," *Journal of Molecular Diagnostics* 11, no. 4 (July 2009): 306–10.

5. Brenda Finucane, Sharyn Lincoln, Lindsay Bailey, and Christa Lese Martin, "Prognostic Dilemmas and Genetic Counseling for Prenatally Detected Fragile X Gene Expansions," *Prenatal Diagnosis* 37 (2017): 37–42.

6. Sarah L. Nolin, Anne Glicksman, Nicole Ersalesi, Carl Dobkin, W. Ted Brown, Ru Cao, Eliot Blatt, et al., "Fragile X Full Mutation Expansions Are Inhibited by One or More AGG Interruptions in Premutation Carriers," *Genetics in Medicine* 17 (2015): 358–64.

7. Sarah Nolin, interview, November 13, 2019.

8. Sarah L. Nolin, Anne Glicksman, Nicole Tortora, Emily Allen, James Macpherson, Montserrat Mila, Angela M. Vianna-Morgante, et al., "Expansions and Contractions of the FMR1 CGG Repeat in 5,508 Transmissions of Normal, Intermediate, and Premutation Alleles," *American Journal of Medical Genetics A* 179, no. 7 (July 2019): 1148–56.

9. Anne-Marie Laberge and Wylie Burke, "Testing Minors for Breast Cancer," *AMA Journal of Ethics, Virtual Mentor* 9, no. 1 (2007): 6–11.

10. Finucane et al., "Prognostic Dilemmas and Genetic Counseling."

11. Amy Cronister, interview, January 22, 2018.

12. Imran S. Haque, Gabriel A. Lazarin, H. Peter Kang, Eric A. Evans, James D. Goldberg, and Ronald J. Wapner, "Modeled Fetal Risk of Genetic Diseases Identified by Expanded Carrier Screening," *Journal of the American Medical Association* 316, no. 7 (2016): 734–42.

13. Kyle A. Beauchamp, Katherine A. Johansen Taber, and Dale Muzzey, "Clinical Impact and Cost-Effectiveness of a 176-Condition Expanded Carrier Screen," *Genetics in Medicine* 21 (2019): 1948–57.

14. American College of Obstetrics and Gynecology, Committee on Genetics, "Carrier Screening in the Age of Genomic Medicine," Committee Opinion, no. 690, March 2017.

15. Ronald J. Wapner and Joseph R. Biggio, "Commentary: Expanded Carrier Screening—How Much Is Too Much?" *Genetics in Medicine* 21 (2019): 1927–30.

16. Josef Ekstein and Howard Katzenstein, "The Dor Yeshorim Story: Community-Based Carrier Screening for Tay-Sachs Disease," *Advances in Genetics* 44 (2001): 297–310.

17. Wapner and Biggio, "Commentary," 1928.

18. Melanie is a pseudonym. Minor details have been changed for anonymity and clarity.

19. Melanie, interview, January 15, 2020.

20. Erica Spiegel, interview, December 16, 2019.

21. Sari Lieberman, Shachar Zuckerman, Ephrat Levy-Lahad, and Gheona Altarescu, "Conflicts Regarding Genetic Counseling for Fragile X Syndrome Screening: A Survey of Clinical Geneticists and Genetic Counselors in Israel," *American Journal of Medical Genetics Part A* 155 (2011): 2154–60.
22. Gil Eyal, Maya Sabatello, Kathryn Tabb, Rachel Adams, Matthew Jones, Frank R. Lichtenberg, Alondra Nelson, et al., "The Physician-Patient Relationship in the Age of Precision Medicine," *Genetics in Medicine* 21, no. 4 (April 2019): 813–15.
23. Susan Lindee, *Moments of Truth in Genetic Medicine* (Baltimore, MD: Johns Hopkins University Press, 2005).
24. David Hessl, interview, September 30, 2015.

8. BORDERLANDS OF THE PREMUTATION

1. Deborah A. Hall, "In the Gray Zone in the Fragile X Gene: What Are the Key Unanswered Clinical and Biological Questions?" *Tremor and Other Hyperkinetic Movements* 4 (2014): 208.
2. Isabel Fernandez-Carvajal, Blanca Lopez Posadas, Ruiqin Pan, Christopher Raske, Paul J. Hagerman, and Flora Tassone, "Expansion of an *FMR1* Grey-Zone Allele to a Full Mutation in Two Generations," *Journal of Molecular Diagnostics* 11, no. 4 (July 2009): 306–10.
3. Hall, "In the Gray Zone."
4. Hall, "In the Gray Zone."
5. Danuta Z. Loesch, Flora Tassone, George D. Mellick, Malcolm Horne, Justin P. Rubio, Minh Q. Bui, David Francis, and Elsdon Storey, "Evidence for the Role of FMR1 Gray Zone Alleles as a Risk Factor for Parkinsonism in Females," *Movement Disorders* 33, no. 7 (July 2018): 1178–81.
6. Atefeh Entezari, Mahmoud Shekari Khaniani, Tayyeb Bahrami, Sima Mansoori Derakhshan, and Hossein Darvish, "Screening for Intermediate CGG Alleles of FMR1 Gene in Male Iranian Patients with Parkinsonism," *Neurological Sciences* 38, no. 1 (January 2017): 123–28.
7. Deborah A. Hall, Sukriti Nag, Bichun Ouyang, David A. Bennett, Yuanqing Liu, Aisha Ali, Lili Zhou, and Elizabeth Berry-Kravis, "Fragile X Gray Zone Alleles Are Associated with Signs of Parkinsonism and Earlier Death," *Movement Disorders* 35, no. 8 (2020): 1448–56.

8. Gülen Eda Utine, Pelin Özlem Şimşek-Kiper, Özlem Akgün-Doğan, Gizem Ürel-Demir, Yasemin Alanay, Dilek Aktaş, Koray Boduroğlu, et al., "Fragile X–Associated Premature Ovarian Failure in a Large Turkish Cohort: Findings of Hacettepe Fragile X Registry," *European Journal of Obstetrics, Gynecology, & Reproductive Biology* 221 (February 2018): 76–80.

9. Marsha R. Mailick, Jinkuk Hong, Paul Rathouz, Mei W. Baker, Jan S. Greenberg, Leann Smith, and Matthew Maenner, "Low-Normal *FMR1* CGG Repeat Length: Phenotypic Associations," *Frontiers in Genetics* 5 (2014): 309.

10. Andrea Weghofer, Muy-Kheng Tea, David H. Barad, Ann Kim, Christian F. Singer, Klaus Wagner, and Norbert Gleicher, "*BRCA1/2* Mutations Appear Embryo-Lethal Unless Rescued by Low (CGG n<26) *FMR1* Sub-Genotypes: Explanation for the 'BRCA Paradox?'" *PLOS ONE* 7, no. 9 (September 12, 2012): e44753.

11. Margaret and Joseph are pseudonyms. Some details have been changed for anonymity and clarity. Margaret was interviewed on October 7, 2016.

12. Julie A. Deisinger, *The Broad Autism Phenotype* (Bingley, UK: Emerald Group, 2015), 1.

13. "Endophenotypes," *Harvard Mental Health Letter*, September 2007.

14. Molly Losh, Deborah Childress, Kristen Lam, and Joseph Piven, "Defining Key Features of the Broad Autism Phenotype: A Comparison Across Parents of Multiple- and Single-Incidence Autism Families," *American Journal of Medical Genetics B: Neuropsychiatric Genetics* 147B, no. 4 (June 5, 2008): 424–33.

15. Deisinger, *The Broad Autism Phenotype*.

16. Wai Chan, Leanne E. Smith, Jan S. Greenberg, Jinkuk Hong, and Marsha R. Mailick, "Executive Function Mediates the Effect of Behavioral Problems on Depression in Mothers of Children with Developmental Disabilities," *American Journal of Intellectual Developmental Disabilities* 122, no. 1 (January 2017): 11–24.

17. Molly Losh, Jessica Klusek, Gary E. Martin, John Sideris, Morgan Parlier, and Joseph Piven, "Defining Genetically Meaningful Language and Personality Traits in Relatives of Individuals with Fragile X Syndrome and Relatives of Individuals with Autism," *American Journal of Medical Genetics B: Neuropsychiatric Genetics* 159B (June 12, 2012): 660–668, 665.

18. Anne C. Wheeler, John Sideris, Randi Hagerman, Elizabeth Berry-Kravis, Flora Tassone, and Donald B. Bailey Jr., "Developmental Profiles

of Infants with an *FMR1* Premutation," *Journal of Neurodevelopmental Disorders* 8 (2016): 40.

19. Sally Clifford, Cheryl Dissanayake, Quang M. Bui, Richard Huggins, Annette K. Taylor, and Danuta Z. Loesch, "Autism Spectrum Phenotype in Males and Females with Fragile X Full Mutation and Premutation," *Journal of Autism and Developmental Disorders* 37 (2007): 738–47.

20. Ivan Iossifov, Michael Ronemus, Dan Levy, Zihua Wang, Inessa Hakker, Julie Rosenbaum, Boris Yamrom, et al., "De Novo Gene Disruptions in Children on the Autism Spectrum," *Neuron* 74 (2012): 285–99.

21. A. Schneider, C. Johnson, F. Tassone, S. Sansone, R.J. Hagerman, E. Ferrer, S.M. Rivera, and D. Hessl, "Broad Autism Spectrum and Obsessive-Compulsive Symptoms in Adults with the Fragile X Premutation," *Clinical Neuropsychology* 30, no. 6 (August 2016): 929–43.

22. Mara, Tommy, and Matt are pseudonyms. Some details have been changed for anonymity and clarity.

23. Randi Hagerman, interview, February 5, 2019.

9. OUTCOMES

1. Laurie, Dan, Mark, Sarah, and Ian are pseudonyms. Some details have been changed for anonymity and clarity. Interviews took place on several occasions between March 26, 2016, and June 15, 2020.

2. Donald Bailey, Robert N. Golden, Jane Roberts, and Amy Ford, "Maternal Depression and Developmental Disability: Research Critique," *Mental Retardation and Developmental Disabilities Research Review* 13, no. 4 (2007): 321 29.

3. Jane E. Roberts, Bridgette L. Tonnsen, Lindsay M. McCary, Amy L. Ford, Robert N. Golden, and Donald B. Bailey Jr., "Trajectory and Predictors of Depression and Anxiety Disorders in Mothers with the FMR1 Premutation," *Biological Psychiatry* 79, no. 10 (May 15, 2016): 850–57.

4. Andrea Schneider, Tri Indah Winarni, Ana María Cabal-Herrera, Susan Bacalman, Louise Gane, Paul Hagerman, Flora Tassone, and Randi Hagerman, "Elevated *FMR1*-mRNA and Lowered FMRP—A Double-Hit Mechanism for Psychiatric Features in Men with *FMR1* Premutations," *Translational Psychiatry* 10, no. 1 (2020): 205.

5. Matthew R. Robinson, Aaron Kleinman, Mariaelisa Graff, Anna A.E. Vinkhuyzen, David Couper, Michael B. Miller, Wouter J. Peyrot, Abdel

Abdellaoui, et al., "Genetic Evidence of Assortative Mating in Humans," *Nature Human Behaviour* 1, no. 1 (2017).

6. J. Purdon Martin and Julia Bell, "A Pedigree of Mental Defect Showing Sex-Linkage," *Journal of Neurology, Neurosurgery & Psychiatry* 6, nos. 3–4 (July 1943): 154–57.

7. Maria J. Aristizabal, Ina Anreiter, Thorhildur Halldorsdottir, Candice L. Odgers, Thomas W. McDade, Anna Goldenberg, Sara Mostafavi, et al., "Biological Embedding of Experience: A Primer on Epigenetics," *Proceedings of the National Academy of Science* 117, no. 38 (September 22, 2020): 23261–69.

8. Verónica Martínez-Cerdeño; Mirna Lechpammer, Aisha Lott, Andrea Schneider, and Randi Hagerman, "Fragile X–Associated Tremor/Ataxia Syndrome in a Man in His 30s," *Journal of the American Medical Association Neurology* 72, no. 9 (September 1, 2015): 1070–73.

9. Randi J. Hagerman, interview, June 8, 2020.

10. Carl F. Weems, Kasey M. Saltzman, Allan L. Reiss, and Victor G. Carrion, "A Prospective Test of the Association Between Hyperarousal and Emotional Numbing in Youth with a History of Traumatic Stress," *Journal of Clinical Child & Adolescent Psychology* 32, no. 1 (March 2003): 166–71.

11. Schneider et al., "Elevated FMR1-mRNA."

12. Jonathan Polussa, Andrea Schneider, and Randi Hagerman, "Molecular Advances Leading to Treatment Implications for Fragile X Premutation Carriers," *Brain Disorders & Therapy* 3 (2014):100011.

13. Anne Skomorowsky, "The Carriers," *Scientific American Mind* 27, no. 2 (March 2016): 34–41.

ACKNOWLEDGMENTS

THE CARRIERS could never have been written without the grace and courage of the many patients and family members I have interviewed over the past six years. While all subjects were eager to contribute whatever information they could for the benefit of others with fragile X disorders, I made a decision to refer to subjects with pseudonyms and to alter recognizable details; in some cases, I have combined or exchanged one individual's details with another's. To the families: you know who you are. I cannot thank you enough for allowing me to learn from you and to tell your stories.

Writing this book would have been impossible without the passion of Randi Hagerman, who helped me as a friend, a fact-checker, and, perhaps most of all, the conduit to the families and researchers I have written about here. She has also been a generous and willing subject and host.

Randi and her husband, Paul Hagerman, were thoughtful early readers of my manuscript, as was Stephanie Sherman, who kindly and tactfully helped me understand fragile X genetics to the extent that I do. For their insights and friendship, I am grateful to Louise Gane, Shalini Kedia, Robby Miller, Larry Nelson, Wilmar Saldarriaga Gil and his family, and Flora Tassone.

I am grateful to the many other clinicians and scientists who shared their knowledge with me, including Don and Pam Bailey, James Bourgeois, Amy Cronister, Jim Grigsby, Deborah Hall, David Hessl, Heather Hipp, Peng Jin, Maureen Leehey, Larry Lipson, Molly Losh, Marsha Mailick, Verónica Martínez-Cerdeño, Daniel Navon, Shivani Nazareth, David Nelson, Sally Nolin, Ben Oostra, Andrea Schneider, Erica Spiegel, Amy Talboy, Laura Yuriko González Teshima, Peter Todd, the late Steve Warren, Jayne Dixon Weber, and Sergio Villada.

My agent, Susan Cohen, took a special interest in my book and devoted herself to it for scant reward. To everyone at Columbia University Press—my editor Miranda Martin, Leslie Kriesel, Gregory McNamee, and Brian Smith—thanks for all your hard work and care. For working with me on my original article, "The Carriers," thanks to Claudia Wallis and Daisy Yuhas.

For their superb editing, I am grateful to Margot Herrera and Lauren Sandler. Lauren, special thanks for your mentorship and vibes. Without you and the staff and my co-fellows at the Op-Ed Project, I would never have had the nerve.

Many others supported me throughout this work, as writers dispensing wisdom, close friends, and often both: Ursula

Abrams, Edward Ball, Hannah Brown, Jennifer Downey, Mike Miller, Sarah Paul, Elizabeth Tillinghast, John Young, and Winnie Chapin Young.

For my mother, Phyllis, my brother, Andrew, and my late father, Peter, I will always be grateful.

Finally, to my husband, Doug, and daughters, Charlotte and Rebecca: you are everything.

INDEX

Note: Names in quotation marks are pseudonyms.

fragile X–associated tremor/ataxia
syndrome (FXTAS) (*continued*)
substance abuse, 33–34; and
treatment, 136–39; and tremors,
7, 27, 35, 110, 123, 125, 147, 148, 181,
219. *See also* "Calvin"; "Clay";
"Corey"; "Dave"; "Lewis";
"Patricia"; "Thomas"
fragile X mental retardation
protein. *See* FMRP
fragile X premutation, vii–x;
anecdotal associations with
medical and psychiatric
conditions, 23, 29–30, 121;
associated conditions
(*see* ADHD; anxiety; arthritis;
ataxia/gait changes; autism;
autoimmune disorders; balance
problems; behavioral symptoms;
bipolar disorder; broad autism
phenotype; chronic fatigue;
chronic pain; depression;
executive dysfunction; fertility
issues; fragile X–associated
neuropsychiatric disorders;
fragile X–associated primary
ovarian insufficiency; fragile
X–associated tremor/ataxia
syndrome; hypertension;
injuries/falls; learning differences; memory impairment;
menopause, early; migraines;
restless legs syndrome; sleep
disorders; social deficits/social
anxiety; tremors); autopsies of
brains of patients with fragile X
premutation, 23, 128–29, 135,
147–48; carrier distress linked to

"midrange" CGG repeat
numbers, 218; carriers as
"patients-in-waiting," 193, 226;
and CGG repeats, 51–53, 73, 82,
126, 196–97 (*see also* CGG
repeats); chance of passing on
full mutation based on number
of CGG repeats, 174–79,
175(table), 177–78(table);
comorbidities, 31, 150, 152–53;
conventional understanding of
carriers as unaffected by carrier
status, 4–5; discovery of
premutation and its effects in the
1990s, 6, 52, 121–23, 195;
EFXN-proposed hierarchy of
fragile X–associated diagnoses,
154; and epigenetics and
victimization, 220–23; female
carriers (*see* female carriers of
fragile X premutation; mothers
of fragile X children or fragile X
premutation carriers); and
FMRP levels, 23, 218–19; and
genetic counseling, 169–93
(*see also* genetic counseling/
family planning; genetic
testing); "gray zone" carriers,
195–212 (*see also* "gray zone"
carriers of fragile X premutation); guilt felt by carriers,
191; Hagermans' studies
(*see* Hagerman, Paul; Hagerman,
Randi); and intellectual
disability, 23, 84; and interplay of
genetics and environment,
144–50; lack of overt deficits in
many carriers, 9–10; male

INDEX

CPSIA information can be obtained
at www.ICGtesting.com
Printed in the USA
BVHW040857190522
637507BV00015B/257/J